ENCYCLOPAEDIA OF
NATURAL HEALTH AND HEALING

ENCYCLOPAEDIA
OF NATURAL HEALTH
AND HEALING

HARVEY DAY

KAYE & WARD · LONDON

First published by
Kaye & Ward Ltd
21 New Street, London EC2M 4NT

Copyright © Kaye and Ward Ltd 1979

ISBN 0 7182 1204 5

Set in VIP Palatino by S. G. Mason (Chester) Ltd.,
Printed in Great Britain by Fakenham Press Limited,
Fakenham, Norfolk

PREFACE

I have written this book to give readers facts about foods and dispel many cherished fallacies.

There are no such comestibles as 'health foods,' which if eaten in quantity will bring about health. All naturally grown foods contribute towards health if eaten in small quantities. The idea that if a food is good, a great deal of it is better does not follow. Too much of any food or vitamin creates an imbalance and may result in more harm than good. There is the well known case in 1974 of Mr Basil Brown, Ph.D. in chemistry, who in ten days swallowed carrot juice containing 70 million units of vitamin A because he thought it was good for him. He turned bright yellow and died of vitamin poisoning. The vitamin rarely kills because it does not become toxic till 100,000 units are taken daily over a long period – but 70 million in 10 days!

Beware of those who enthuse about 'wonder foods' such as wheat germ, honey, yogurt, food yeast and molasses. Each is beneficial if taken in moderation but harmful in excess. Wheat germ was so boosted as a wonder food in 1972 that many Olympic athletes stuffed themselves with it without improving their performances one whit. Many believe that wheat germ and honey improve sexual ability and the Japanese bought honey in such quantities that all they did was to send up the price. Yogurt is supposed to increase longevity but Metchnikoff, the great advocate of yogurt, died at 71. Yeast is a fine protein food but if more than half an ounce a day is eaten a strain is thrown on the kidneys. Too much molasses fattens.

As for vitamins, they are not foods but accessory factors, and the best sources are fresh fruit and vegetables, grown in compost. Where the diet is unbalanced or there is illness, due in almost all instances to faulty diet, the appropriate vitamins may be taken, but not indiscriminately, as so many people do.

An experiment was carried out in America to discover whether additional vitamins made people fitter. Capsules of synthetic vitamins A, B₁, B₂, and C were given to 1,242 children and 214 adults in addition to their normal diet, but were found to have little effect. The same vitamins were also given to school children in Ipswich, Glossop and London and, according to the *BMJ** 'The vitamins had no significant effect on the rate of growth, muscular strength, condition of the teeth and gums, or absence from school on account of illness.'

Used judiciously, however, vitamins can be of value, but so many people swallow so many vitamin pills daily that they must rattle when they walk and the only people to benefit are the manufacturers and the advertising agencies.

I believe that vegetarianism will result in sound health *if the diet is balanced* but I know vegetarians who are sickly because they know nothing about the art of eating. Too many nuts and protein foods can cause indigestion; an overload of starches can result in constipation, pimples and boils as well as headaches.

Beware of cranks and converts to vegetarianism. Proselytes are usually the most rabid of all and are apt to regard meat and all processed foods as 'poison.' Yet commonsense should tell them that millions eat meat, white bread, white·sugar, etc., and to all appearances seem healthy enough. Some even live to be centenarians. So to all who read this book I urge tolerance and moderation.

Remember that foods, vitamins and herbs do not *cure* disease. Nature alone does that. If left to itself the body has tremendous powers of recuperation. Often a rest and a fast can achieve more than doctors with strings of degrees after their names. Dr William Evans says† that when he became House Physician to Sir John Parkinson he was told that except for emergencies patients admitted should not be given medicines or tablets until he had seen them the following morning. When after a night's rest Parkinson visited them many showed such improvement that no further medical care was necessary. This was a lesson he never forgot. If a patient demanded medicine he was given a placebo and, he recalls, 'The healing property of coloured water has truly amazed me!'

A balanced diet, fresh air and sunshine, hydrotherapy, acupuncture, homeopathy, osteopathy, chiropractic, herbs and exercise merely assist the healing process till complete health is attained.

*British Medical Journal.
†*Journey to Harley Street.*

In all things use common sense, though why it is so named I do not know as it is one of the rarest of all qualities. Victor Hugo said: 'Common sense is in spite of, not the result of, education.'

It is fashionable to criticise the NHS which, for all its imperfections is an imaginative conception which has raised the level of health in Britain, and the GPs and nurses, the backbone of the service, are generally speaking, devoted to the care of the sick.

American medicine compares unfavourably with the NHS, for according to a Report issued by the AMA* in 1974, more than 2,380,000 needless operations were performed, resulting in 11,900 deaths at a cost to patients of £2,000,000,000. A woman going into hospital for blood tests, for instance, was asked to pay £60 in advance; the parents of a child who suffered a hairline fracture while doing a cartwheel were charged £50 for a plaster cast and thought they had got off lightly. No self-respecting doctor earns less than 50,000 dollars a year and a major operation can cripple a family financially, even though the patient may be insured.

Those who criticise our system should think, not of ways to destroy it, but to improve and cut costs, for we take advantage of the system because it is free. A Report issued by the Office of Health Economics stated that too many patients received costly treatment for ailments they could well treat themselves. A woman admitted to the Radcliffe Infirmary, Oxford, for instance, who complained of bizarre symptoms ranging from headache to palpitations was given a series of tests over a 16-day period which cost £160. Only after the tests proved negative was it found that she was taking tablets originally prescribed for her asthma!

Millions clutter up surgeries all over the country for trivial complaints and few are satisfied unless they leave 'with a bottle of something' or a box of tablets. A neighbour of mine boasted about the cost of his treatment as if it were a status symbol. 'I was given a box of 20 tablets which cost £7!' implying that others whose drugs cost less were inferior.

Dr James Struthers of the Ministry of Health complained in 1964 that £4,800,000 a year was spent on prescriptions that did little or no good, and Professor Bryan that '£100,000,000 is spent each year on dispensing drugs from doctors' prescriptions when £20,000,000 would do.'

In the same year Dr Powell Evans of Wimbledon was quoted as saying: 'The most vital instrument in the doctor's surgery is the dust bin. It is needed to take the constant flow of drug-makers'

*American Medical Association

publicity hand-outs and samples. The flood has become an attempt to distort the doctors' judgement of the right treatment. This unnecessary advertising is possible only through the fortunes the firms are making through the NHS.'*

In Russia, which is not the Shangri-La that some people imagine, private practice is illegal and there are more doctors, 85% of them women, per head of the population than in any other country. Generally they are overworked and underpaid.

Professor Nikolai Amosoff, Director of Kiev Institute of Pectoral Surgery and recipient of the coveted Lenin Prize, stated: 'Disease is not a normal part of man's physiological make-up. . . Man is responsible for his health. He can preserve and restore it by his own sometimes difficult efforts. Women live longer than men. This is not predestined by hereditary factors or biological reasons; alcohol, tobacco, early retirement, inactivity and excessive food are undoubtedly causing this disparity.

Man's irresponsibility towards his own health is stimulated by such seeming blessings as the discovery of new medicinal agents and the general success of medical science. This leads to the groundless belief in "miracle drugs" and techniques, and the lessening of the physical and particularly psychological faculty of the body to resist and correct, organic malfunctions.'

What we need today is a service that will prevent people from falling ill, rather than letting them fall ill and then trying to cure them. GPs are so overworked that they haven't the time for preventative medicine, and if they tried, patients would leave them with the speed of lemmings leaping off the cliffs of Norway. This book gives readers some of the knowledge they need to guide them towards health.

*Herald: 12.6.1961

Cross referencing by the use of italics has been included where it is felt that the reader might wish to refer to another entry for further information.

Dorchester-on-Thames
Oxfordshire

A

A Vitamin. See Vitamin A.

Acid. Term applied to any food which has a sharp or sour taste, in chemistry substances which turn blue litmus paper red are called acids. The majority of acids which contain oxygen are known as oxyacids; those not containing oxygen are termed hydrogen acids or hydracids.

Acid Base. When the metallic elements present in foods are oxidised in the body they give rise to bases, and when sulphur and phosphorus in foods are oxidised they give rise to fixed acids; viz., sulphuric and phosphoric acids. Both bases and acids are excreted in the urine, the reaction of the urine depending on the predominance of one or the other. Meat, which is mainly protein, produces acid end products; fruits (even the very acid ones) produce basic end products, and are called alkaline. For sound health there should be a balance in which vegetables and fruits predominate.

Fruit acids are composed of carbon, hydrogen and oxygen and differ from the products of decomposition and oxidation such as butyric acid, sulphuric acid, phosphoric acid, uric acid, etc., which are the results of a high protein diet. The fruit and vegetable acids are citric, gallic, malic, oxalic, tannic and tartaric. Lactic acid occurs in milk products and formic acid in honey.

The following foods have an acid base: bacon, bread (white more than wholemeal), cheese, cobnuts, oatmeal, eggs, haddock, peanuts, peas, pork, rice, beef, steak and walnuts, to name only a few.

Foods with an alkaline base are: almonds, apples, bananas, Brazil nuts, Brussels sprouts, butter beans, cabbage, carrots, cauliflowers, celery, plain chocolate, cocoa, currants, lemon, lime, grapefruit, lettuce, whole milk, skimmed milk, onions, garlic, oranges, potatoes, prunes, rhubarb, tomatoes, turnips and many other vegetables and fruits.

These lists have been taken at random and in order to maintain normal good health the diet should contain a preponderance of alkaline base foods.

Acorn. No longer considered edible in Britain though during the nomadic stages and for centuries after, acorns were used as food. Throughout the Mediterranean coastal regions the acorn of the Holm Oak (*Quercus ilex*) is still eaten. In parts of Spain and Portugal they command the same price as chestnuts and when boiled have a sweet, nutty flavour. In Algeria and Morocco they are roasted in ashes or boiled, and in Turkey they are first buried in the earth, then washed, ground and dried and, with the addition of sugar and spice, made into a popular dish called *racahout*.

In North America where there are 60 species of oak, acorns have always been eaten by the Indians, who grind them into a fine meal which is worked into a dough and baked into bread and cakes. John Muir, a pioneer who explored the mountains of California, found acorn cakes and bread to be compact, strengthening foods. Dried acorns contain 4.10% water, 8.10% protein, 48.00% carbohydrates, 37.40% fat and 2.40% mineral salts, especially rich in potassium.

Acupuncture. One of the oldest forms of healing known, for details of acupuncture treatment occur in *Nei Ching* (The Yellow Emperor's Classic of Internal Medicine) written about the year 400 BC, which is the foundation of all Chinese medicine. The treatment is carried out by inserting fine needles into one or more of some 800 points in the body. It operates on the principle that the vital force or Ch'i energy, circulates from one organ to another along channels called meridians, always following a set route. Unless this energy flows freely and in the correct strength one or more of the organs will not function efficiently, and treatment by needles is used to restore the vital force Ch'i (pronounced Kee). Correct manipulation of the needles draws the energy to an organ, disperses from it, drains it, etc.

Diagnosis is carried out by finding out the history of the disease, symptoms, etc.; by listening to the sound of the voice and what is said; by observing mechanical defects, colour of the skin, posture, etc.; by judging the texture of the skin, variation of temperature of skin surface and the feeling of the twelve pulses on the wrists – six on either wrist.

Many other factors are taken into consideration: the seasons, moon phases, time of the day, emotional and mental state of the patient, and body smell. As this has to be thorough, an initial consultation may take from two to four hours.

Diet is important for the body to function properly and general rules are that white sugar should be replaced by either brown sugar or honey (not more than four tablespoons of honey should be taken daily); white flour products should be replaced by wholewheat grown preferably in compost; salads and fresh fruit should predominate; vegetables should be lightly cooked; condiments, sauces, pickles and chutnies should be eaten sparingly or cut out altogether; tinned foods should not be eaten; processed foods or foods treated with chemicals should be avoided; and moderation in all things should be observed.

Moxabustion is also used in acupuncture. Once derided and opposed by the medical profession, acupuncture is now accepted by the West, is widely used by doctors in France and Germany, is gaining ground in Britain, and breaking down prejudice in America. It has been used effectively as an anaesthetic under which major operations have been performed, with the patients conscious, taking nourishment and aware of all that is going on; and there have been no unpleasant after effects, such as ordinary anaesthetics produce. Needless to say acupuncture is not successful in all cases, but neither is allopathy. Acupuncture has, however, been successful very often, where orthodox medicine has failed. See: Moxabustion.

Acupuncture Association. A charity, the objects of which are: (1) to promote and encourage the study and knowledge of acupuncture (2) to establish the status, regulate the conduct, and protect the interests of practitioners of acupuncture so as to promote and maintain in the public interest proper standards for the practice of acupuncture (3) to establish, maintain and publish a register of qualified acupuncturists and to promote honourable practice (4) to exclude malpractice and to decide all questions of professional conduct and etiquette among practising acupuncturists, etc. The Chairman is Sidney Rose-Neil and the address of the London Office is: 34 Alderney Street, London SW1V 4EU. Telephone (01) 834 1012. In America; The Acupuncture Medical Association of America, 7535 Laurel Canyon Blvd., North Hollywood, CA 91605. Telephone (213) 877-9475.

Acupuncture Clinic, The. A faculty of the College of Chinese Acupuncture (UK), presided over by Professor J. R. Worsley. The address of the Clinic is: Oaken Holt, Farmoor, Oxford OX2 9NY. See: Worsley.

Aykroyd, MD, Dr W. R. Director of the Nutrition Institute, Indian Research Fund Association, Coonoor; Member of the

Health Section of the League of Nations (1931-1935); a pioneer of the science of nutrition; collaborated with *M.K.* (Mahatma *Gandhi* to find cheap and nutritious foods for the Indian people. Author of *Nutrition and Diet* as well as technical books and articles.

Agar-agar. A word derived from the Malaysian to describe an East Indian seaweed from which a gelatinous substance is extracted for use in soups, and as jellies, and is added to a thousand-and-one edibles, and in face creams, toothpastes, etc. It is used as a medium in which to grow cultures. Agar-agar is also an effective natural laxative. The birds' nests used in birds'-nest soup, a Chinese delicacy, are composed mainly of this weed.

Air baths. *Air, light* and *sun* are three great natural healers. Siegert said: 'Air is the bread of the lungs; it cleanses our blood, feeds our tissues, and on which all our vital processes depend. It is also food for the skin, the function of the latter being to absorb pure, strengthening air, as much as to excrete morbid matter and the change of matter products'; and Simon said: 'A better medicine, a more strengthening and nourishing remedy than the atmospheric air, in its purest, unmixed form, does not exist.' See: Muller and Rikli.

Alcohol. Alcohol is generated in wines, spirits and beers during fermentation caused by the action of sugar on yeast. The amount of alcohol varies with different beverages, the consumption of which can be either beneficial or harmful, depending on the amount consumed. Alcohol is not a stimulant but a narcotic. Its chief virtue is that it dulls the higher centres of the brain, removes self-consciousness and worry, soothes the anxious mind and is an aid to sociability. It does not warm the body, but cools it; the feeling of warmth is temporary and illusory, caused by blood being drawn to the surface of the skin, where the heat is soon dissipated. The only reason for indulging in alcoholic beverages is that you like them, when they should be consumed in strictly limited quanties as over-indulgence damages the heart, liver and kidneys, bringing a host of diseases in its train. The food value of alcohol is negligible.

Alexander, Frederick Mathias (1869-1955). Born in Wynyard, Tasmania, where his grand-father owned a large property including Table Cape. As his parents had ample means he spent his childhood in country pursuits and the training and management of horses. At 17 he started work with the Mount

Bischoff Tin Mining Co., where his main interest lay in teaching himself to play the violin and taking part in amateur dramatics. Three years later he went to stay with his uncle James in Melbourne and, with £500 he had saved, spent three months in seeing all that was best in the theatres, art galleries, and then decided to train as a Reciter. He tried a number of jobs in order to pay his way: in an estate agency, a department store and a tea estate and occupied

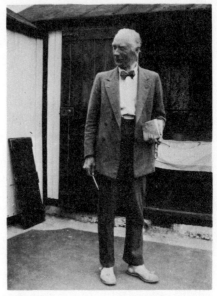

Mathias Alexander

his spare time acting and producing plays. Despite trouble with his vocal organs he was a success. He set about trying to find a way to cure his disability, a full account of his research appearing in *The Use Of The Self.* After he was cured he continued to give recitals and teach others to improve their voices. Then a friend, Dr McKay, urged him to go to London and teach his unique method.

His methods were instantly successful and he numbered among his pupils Henry Irving, Viola Tree, Lily Langtry, Constance Collier, Ascar Asche and Matheson Lang and as a result of his teaching experience wrote *Man's Supreme Inheritance.* Between 1914-1924 he spent half his time in America and half in Britain and produced two more books: *Conscious Control* and *Constructive Conscious Control Of the Individual,* which contained a preface by John Dewey, the American philosopher. These were followed by *The Universal Constant In Living.*

Though Alexander was extremely successful he had a constant struggle for recognition by the medical profession, many of whose members benefited from his teachings. He was a skilled and inspired teacher and Sir Stafford Cripps, who benefited considerably from 'the Alexander Technique', was guest of

5

honour at a dinner to celebrate his 80th birthday and the founding of a Society of Teachers who now carry on his work. Alexander died while still actively at work but his methods survive and fortunately, those who wish to train in his methods can take a three-year course in the Alexander Technique.

Alexander Principle, The. The Alexander Principle is based on the fact that most people misuse their bodies, mainly the neck, by holding and carrying themselves badly and, as the neck, which sits on the spinal column, is a very important part of the human structure, its misuse can affect a multitude of limbs and organs, resulting in a host of pathological conditions: headaches, rheumatism, arthritis and other deep-seated troubles which escape diagnosis by the average medical practitioner. The Alexander Technique teaches one how to balance the body correctly, for posture is all-important; how to sit, stand and hold the body correctly. It teaches people how to do all these things naturally so that the spine and neck are correctly aligned, the feet properly placed as one walks and the body is at all times in a state of balance and relaxation.

The sheer simplicity of the principle has done more to defeat its teachers than anything, for the medical profession could not believe that a principle so simple could have such outstanding results. The Society of The Teachers Of The Alexander Technique has its headquarters at 3 Albert Court, Kensington Gore, London SW7.

Allergy. Derived from the Greek, other, different; and work. It means altered energy; altered reactivity and altered capacity to react; hypersensitivity. An allergen is a substance or condition which generates or produces an allergy. Allergen includes all allergic excitants; that is, anything which excites or produces allergy. A person with an allergy is said to be allergic.

Allergies are not organic diseases like heart disease, tuberculosis or an abcess on the liver but are caused by the body's hypersensitivity to some external cause, such as pollen which bring out rashes. When all other treatment has failed an allergy often responds to hypnotic suggestion.

Allinson, Dr T. R. (1858-1918). Born in Hume, Manchester. At 15 he was disinherited by his step-father and left home with £5 to work as a chemist's assistant. While sometimes working 16 hours a day he read chemistry and medicine, observed how the poor lived and what they ate. When 16, his mother lent him the money to enter Edinburgh University where he read medicine and passed with honours. He did not accept everything he was taught but learnt to think for himself. He studied in Paris and on his return helped in a country practice. Then he went to London where, with his qualifications he could have put up his plate in the West End, but he chose to become a police surgeon, public vaccinator and parish doctor among the needy in Shoreditch, where he worked throughout the small-pox epidemic of 1880-81, gaining valuable experience.

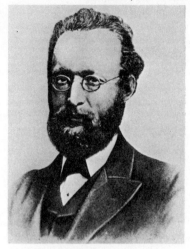

Dr. T. R. Allinson

He discovered that the diet of the poor consisted of tea siftings brewed or boiled; white bread adulterated with bone dust, talcum power, chalk and alum; and butcher's offals, often from diseased animals. To help his patients he experimented with cheap wholesome ingredients: wholewheat bread made with yeast, cottonseed oil instead of butter, cocoa without milk, etc., and to convince them he lived on the diet he prescribed. In 1883 he set up his own surgery, which was always packed, and induced local bakers to make 100% wholewheat loaves from wheat grown in compost, according to his recipe, and gave them gilt certificates signed by him to hang in their windows. By 1890 there were 9,000 bakers making Allinson loaves.

To prove that good health could be maintained cheaply he lived for a period on 6d a day and in a month increased his weight by 3¼ lbs! To demonstrate his theories he gave a three-course supper to 150 women working for charitable associations, at a total cost of 37/6d – or 3d a head. He showed that it was possible to eat well without sacrificing physical efficiency, and at the end of the meal distributed pamphlets containing specimen recipes.

He gave up prescribing drugs, urged his patients to become vegetarians and attacked the medical profession so fiercely in articles and pamphlets that in 1891 he was struck off the register of his college. He took them to court and proved his case, but the

7

Almond

College maintained that it was a 'closed body' with the right to do as it pleased. The case cost him £1,000 but brought him ten times that amount in publicity. Thereafter he described himself as Ex-LRCP, etc., and continued hammering the medical profession. Today all the ideas he advocated have been adopted by food reformers and dieticians and, with much reluctance by many of the medical profession.

Almond. An excellent high-alkaline protein food consisting of

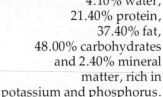

4.10% water,
21.40% protein,
37.40% fat,
48.00% carbohydrates
and 2.40% mineral
matter, rich in
potassium and phosphorus.

Aluminium. Traces of aluminium are to be found in the lungs, heart, kidneys, pancreas and testicles. It is present in fruits, vegetables and meat in microscopic quantities as aluminium oxide or alumina, and its chemical action is similar to that of *magnesium.* Though it has long been suspected that food cooked in aluminium vessels causes cancer and other diseases, especially of the stomach and kidneys, the Mayo Clinic reported that: 'Aluminium cooking utensils do not impart any undesirable qualities to the food prepared in them,' and tests carried out in the laboratory of *The Lancet* proved that the amount dissolved when cooking bland foods was negligible and that acid foods dissolved only traces of aluminium; it is undesirable, nevertheless, to cook highly salted foods, or foods to which soda is added, in aluminium utensils, and food reformers avoid doing so.

Aneurin. Known as *aneurin* in Britain and *thiamin* in America. See: Vitamin B1.

Antibiotics. The word antibiotic did not exist until 1940 when it was coined after the discovery of penicillin. The first antibiotic was actinomycin (1940); clavacin, fumigacin and streptothricin (1942); streptomycin (1943); hrisein (1946); neomycin (1949); streptocin and fradicin (1950); ehrlichin (1951) and canicidin (1952).

Antibiotics are substances that kill harmful bacteria within the body but unfortunately internal bacteria often grow resistant to antibiotics; antibiotics sometimes have harmful side effects and there are people who are allergic to them.

The body has its own enzyme system to defend itself against germs: lysozyme in tears; fibrinogen for clotting blood when the skin is broken or cut; leucocytes, macrophages, etc., which destroy germs if the resistance of the body has not been lowered. Dr T. K. Day of Guy's Hospital London carried out an experiment to find out whether local antibiotics and injected antibiotics were more effective than merely cleaning and disinfecting wounds before they were sutured. He divided 160 patients into three groups: two were treated either with an injection of penicillin or locally applied tetracyline; the third received no antibiotics.

A week later the wounds were examined by a doctor who did not know which method of treatment had been given. He found that the frequency of infection in the two groups treated by antibiotics was *three times* the rate of the group not treated. Cleansing the wounds is most important but this and other experiments have proved that antibiotics interfere with the body's ability to produce disease-fighting antibodies.

Antiseptics. The wide and indiscriminate use of powerful antiseptics is to be deplored for the body has its own germ-fighting mechanisms. See: Soap, Skin.

Apple. Round, firm, fleshy fruit of a *Rosaceous* tree *(Pyrus Malus)* found all over the world in temperate zones. The British apple is probably the descendant of the crab apple which flourished long before the Roman occupation. Norsemen believed it to be the rejuvenating food of the gods and legend has it that the goddess Iduna kept a box of apples for the purpose of giving the gods new life. Once forbidden by most physicians the apple is now known to cure acute cases of stomach and intestinal catarrh if finely grated and eaten raw. It swells in the intestine and the spongy mass absorbs elements that cause irritation. The pectin applied to open wounds heals them rapidly.

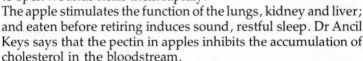

The apple stimulates the function of the lungs, kidney and liver; and eaten before retiring induces sound, restful sleep. Dr Ancil Keys says that the pectin in apples inhibits the accumulation of cholesterol in the bloodstream.

There are 22,000 varieties of apples but none superior in

flavour to the Cox, Russet, Charles Ross or Blenheim though excellent apples are also grown in France, Germany, Australia, New Zealand and the United States. Cooking apples have a far higher acid content than eaters and though most trees bear fruit for only 20 or 30 years varieties have been found in South Kirghizia that have borne fruit for 250 years! One tree had 267 annular rings. A good average eating apple contains 84.80% water, 0.40% protein, 0.50% fat, 13.00% carbohydrates, 0.50% mineral salts, rich in potassium and sodium, and vitamins A, B_1, B_2, and C.

Apple Cider Vinegar. Popularised by Dr D. C. Jarvis, MD, in his books *Folk Medicine* and *Arthritis and Folk Medicine,* in which he claimed to have cured colds, influenza, sinusitis, hay fever and arthritis by regular doses of apple cider vinegar. Though he encountered tremendous opposition and criticism from the medical profession in America, his books have sold by the hundred thousand in the USA and in Britain and thousands have testified that they have been cured by following his advice.

Arsenic. One of the trace elements found in the body in minute quantities, and in animals and vegetables and fruit. The French chemist Bertrand, after many experiments, arrived at the conclusion that arsenic is a constant element of the living cell. Among other foods it is present in peach stones and in egg, the yolk containing twice as much as the albumen. In 1900 Dr Gautier of Paris, found that traces of arsenic are to be found in the epidermis, hair, glands, brain and breast and in a few organs. It is possible, by taking gradually increasing doses, such as the women of Kashmir do to gain pale complexions, eventually to imbibe enough arsenic to kill a man, with complete immunity to themselves.

Arthritis. An obstruction in the body of acid and waste materials caused by faulty diet which clogs the system with uric acid and other poisons, which the liver, kidneys and bladder are unable to throw off. The joints become enlarged, tender and extremely painful and sometimes so stiff that it is impossible to move them. Orthodox medicine falls back on pain-killing drugs and operations during the worst stages, and plastic ball-and-socket joints are provided to replace bone that has been removed.

Dr Aschner the Austrian specialist, and others, have wrought 'miracle' cures by rubbing the affected parts with a pustulant to produce an artificial rash, which brought poisons to the surface and got rid of them, and so cured or relieved even patients in advanced stages of the disease. Remarkable cures have also been obtained by *homeopathy, acupuncture, herbal medicines, osteopathy, chiropractic, fasting* and *naturopathy.* In every instance the diet must be reformed to counteract the effects of faulty living, otherwise the cause will not be removed and arthritis will recur.

Aschner, MD, Dr Bernard. Celebrated Austrian physician who, while practising orthodox medicine kept an open mind and did not hesitate to incorporate any form of healing which cured disease, even if used only by 'quacks'. He has described some effective though unorthodox methods in *The Art Of The Healer,* written for the layman.

Ascorbic Acid. See: Vitamin C.

Aspirin. The most common of all drugs. Belongs to a group of drugs known as salicyclates, the original member of which was obtained from the willow whose botanical name is *Salix.* Willow bark has been used for centuries to cure fevers and rheumatism. Both Hippocrates and Galen prescribed it. Its use by the medical profession, however, dates from 1763 when the Rev. Edward Stone drew the attention of the scientific world to the willow and a century later Dr Maclagan of Glasgow used the bark to treat rheumatism. The active principle, salicin, was isolated and extracted, its chemical structure determined, and derivatives extracted. The most successful, acetylsalicylic acid, was introduced by the Beyer Company of Germany under the trade mark Aspirin; A to denote the acetyl group of atoms and 'sprin' from the botanical genus *Spiraea.*

No one knows how aspirin acts or the exact mechanism by which it relieves pain. Though aspirin alleviates pain it does not cure and the danger of taking aspirin regularly is that it is habit forming, bigger doses have to be taken which cause side effects, internal haemorrhage and even poisoning. Few realise that it is a drug on which one can become 'hooked', and it should never be given indiscriminately to children.

Atherosclerosis. Hardening of the arteries caused by changes in the walls of the arteries, leading to loss of elasticity accompanied by irregular thickening of the artery wall, which narrows the space inside. Muscle and elastic connecting tissue are replaced by a yellow fatty material called cholesterol. Hardening of the arteries usually starts in the forties but there is no need for alarm as it is one of the gradual processes of increasing age. Faulty diet, lack of exercise and worry tend to accelerate hardening of

11

the arteries and bring about premature old age. But the right diet, ample exercise and the cultivation of a placid mind have enabled many to live free from atherosclerosis to 80, 90 and even 100. The idea that the consumption of butter and other animals fats is responsible for the formation of cholesterol has been refuted by the biochemist Dr. Fred Kummerov, adviser to the USA Heart Association. It is only one of the contributory causes.

Aura, The Human. An emanation of one or more of the seven principles of Man, projecting from several inches to two or three feet beyond the body and visible only to those with a highly developed psychic power, though a few with inferior 'sight' can see grosser manifestations of the aura. Auras, which are body-radiations, vary in colour which is said to depend on the nature, character and state of health of the subject, and change as health and mental attitudes change. That auras do exist was first proved by Dr Kilner of St Thomas's Hospital, London, who devised his dycyanin screen consisting of 2 plates of glass ⅛ inch apart, the space being filled with an alcoholic solution of dycyanin, through which the human aura became visible. Within the last 40 years the Kirlians have done some amazing research on the subject, by means of an apparatus to take 'energy photographs' without the use of camera or lens.

Austin, Major Reginald, RAMC. After practising orthodox medicine for years in the Army Austin forsook allopathy for *Naturopathy* and cured hundreds by fasting coupled with a vegetarian diet. His first patient under the new regime was his wife, who was about to undergo an operation for appendicitis. On the day of the operation he whisked her away and restored her to health by fasting, water, and diet. During the First World War he was given charge of a wing of typhoid patients in a hospital in Brighton; he accepted on the understanding that he could use his own methods. Whereas many patients in other wards succumbed, none of his died.

After the war he set up in practice in Duke Street, London, W1, where patients whom orthodox methods had failed to cure flocked to him. He cured a number of people suffering from cancer whose doctors had given them up as incurable, by prolonged fasts, water, fruit juices and a reformed diet. He and *Stanley Lief* were among the pioneers of weight reduction by fasting at a time when doctors believed that fasting was fatal. Austin reduced his own weight from 18 stone to 11 and though medical colleagues ridiculed him they are adopting his ideas 40 years later. Shortly before the Second World War, when he was 70, he undertook an experimental fast of 30 days without ceasing to run his practice. He died during the war, mainly from overwork. See: Lief.

Avocado Pear. A native fruit of regions including Mexico, Colombia and Venezuela. Discovered by Martin Fernandez de Encisco in 1509, who mentioned it in *Suma de Geografia* in 1536. The name avacado is a corruption of the Spanish *aguacate* which is derived from the Aztec *ahuacati*.

The tree grows to a height of 100 feet, but under cultivation to only 30 feet. There are three main varieties: the Mexican which is the hardiest; the West Indian, the largest; and the Guatamalean, which has a thicker rind and a woodier texture. It is grown in many tropical and semi-tropical countries and is rarely attacked by insects or affected by disease. It contains nine vitamins but is especially rich in A and C; 70.55% water, 2.10% protein, 20.00% fat, 6.00% carbohydrates, and 1.35% mineral matter, mainly potassium and sodium. The fruit should be eaten raw as it becomes sour when cooked. It cannot be frozen or chilled successfully and if not eaten at once should not be placed in a refrigerator. It is ready for eating if, when placed in the palms and pressed gently, it yields.

B

B Vitamins. See: Vitamin B_1, B_2, etc.

Bach, Dr Edward, LRCP, MB, MS, DPH (Camb), (1886-1936). A Welshman born in Moseley, near Birmingham. Graduated at Birmingham University and qualified in medicine at University College Hospital, London. Was inspired by *Hahnemann* and turned to *homeopathy* and was eventually appointed pathologist and bacteriologist at the London Homeopathic Hospital, now the Royal.

He realised that disease was not due to physical causes but had its origin in the mind, so advised: 'Treat the patient's personality.' After much research he concluded that there are 38 outstanding states of mind from which the sick suffer, and if

13

banished, health will return. He observed plants, noted the soil in which they grew, the colour and shape of their petals, whether they were propagated by tuber, root or seed, and a host of other details. He was strongly psychic, 'felt' that the vibrations emitted by flowers contained healing elements more potent than those from any other part of the plant, and devised an entirely new form of healing. Being hypersensitive he could place his palms over the petals and feel the vibrations they sent out. If he placed a bloom in the palm of his hand or on his tongue he could feel in his body the effects of the properties it possessed. Some petals vitalised; others caused pain, brought on fevers, produced rashes or even made him vomit. After countless experiments he devised, by trial and error, a method of potentising his remedies and wrote *Heal Thyself*, the first of many books outlining his theories. He travelled throughout England and Wales collecting plants and describing their properties. His ideas were ridiculed by the medical profession and when he wrote articles proclaiming that his methods could cure he was warned that he was advertising and would be struck off the Register if he did not desist. So convinced was he, however, that his form of treatment, which had put scores of 'incurables' on their feet, was sound, that he defied the GMC, who decided it was better to ignore him than take action.

Bach obtained such astonishing results that soon other colleagues rallied to him and learnt how to apply the Bach remedies, and today there are Bach practitioners in every continent, many of them medical men.

Bacteria. Derived from the Greek *bakteria*, rod, because of their shape; known under various names such as *bacilli, cocci, spirella*, etc.; microbes, germs. Extremely minute living organisms, whether plant or animal, existing throughout nature, in water, air and in all foods. Though the word is usually associated with disease and fermentation, most germs are harmless and indeed, serve useful functions in the body, where they act on proteins, fats and carbohydrates; on fats they act as lipase (an enzyme of pancreatic and gastric juices) and produce lower acids (valeric, butyric, etc.) and their action also enables the body to manufacture certain vitamins, such as C and B_{12}.

The bacteria of disease will never attack healthy tissue and the resistance of the body must in some way have been lowered to enable them to undermine the body and cause disease; and as even the healthiest of humans are sometimes 'off colour', all are apt to fall prey to bacteria at some time.

That even deadly bacteria will not affect a healthy body was proved by 150 experiments between 1914 and 1918 undertaken by Dr John B. Fraser, MD. Between 1911-1913 the single point 'When Does The Germ Appear?' was studied, and the answer was: 'After the onset of disease'. This led to the supposition that germs were simply by-products of disease, and possibly harmless.

The first experiment was made in 1914 when a group of citizens in Toronto undertook to swallow virulent germs in order to prove that they would not harm healthy bodies. In the first experiment 50,000 diphtheria germs were swallowed in a glass of water, the reason for choosing these germs was that in aconite they had a reliable remedy, which lessened risk. In the second experiment millions of diphtheria germs were swabbed over the tonsils, soft palate and under the tongue, and in neither case was this followed by the disease. In the third test pneumonia germs were swallowed in milk, water, bread, meat, etc., and persistent efforts were made to coax them to develop, again without success. Then typhoid germs were taken in unpasteurised milk, water, meat, potatoes, bread, fish, etc., but the disease failed to appear. Finally a series of similar tests were made with the dreaded meningitis germs, with no harmful results.

On one occasion during this period the famous Viennese physician Dr Pettenknofer, startled a class of students by picking up a tumbler of water containing millions of cholera bacilli, and swallowing the contents. He did not die or even contract the disease. And Dr Thomas Powell, who died of natural causes in his 80th year, time and again challenged his colleagues to produce a single disease in his body by germ innoculation. He was even innoculated with the germs of bubonic plague! This proved to Dr Fraser and those who took part in the experiments that for germs to take and flourish, a suitable tissue must exist. As a result he wrote an article entitled 'The Germs Cause Disease' which was printed in *Physical Culture*, May 1919.

Banana. The name of this fruit was derived from the Congolese and was adopted by the Portuguese. Centuries earlier it was known in India as a the fruit of the Tree of the Knowledge of Good and Evil and when introduced into Rome it was called *Musa Sapientum*, Fruit of the Wise Men. Though originally a tropical fruit, it also flourishes in semi-tropical regions and is

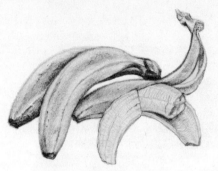

eaten the world over. It is one of the finest of all fruits as it can be digested by all and is especially suitable for infant-feeding, in malnutrition and reducing diets, nephritic diets, for combating acidosis, preventing deficiency diseases, and for intestinal disturbances. It is often the only food that can be digested by victims of celiac disease and anorexia. As it is mildly laxative and the carbohydrate is quickly assimilated it is ideal for the prospective mother and her infant.

If stored, the unripe banana will gradually ripen and eventually the carbohydrate will be converted almost entirely into easily digested fruit sugars. The skin of a fully ripe banana is richly flecked with brown, and in this condition the fruit consists of 75.30% water, 1.30% protein, 0.60% fat, 22.00% carbohydrates, and 0.80% mineral matter, being especially rich in potassium. It also contains vitamins A, B, C and G. Bananas and skimmed milk may form the basis of an efficient and well balanced reducing diet.

Barker, Sir Herbert Atkinson (1869-1950). Son of a solicitor and county coroner in South Lancashire who, because of ill health, was sent to Canada to recuperate on a farm. On the voyage he put into place a passenger's elbow that had been dislocated in an accident and in Canada he enjoyed considerable success in replacing the displaced joints of farm hands and animals. On his return to England he joined his cousin, Robert Atkinson, in his bone-setting practice. Both came from a race of yeoman farmers who had practised bone-setting for more than 200 years.

After a year Barker set up on his own in Manchester where he gained the respect and friendship of Walter Whitehead, Professor of Clinical Medicine at the University. Gradually he built up a practice mainly among footballers and athletes in the North and, though some doctors were hostile, many sent him patients. After 16 years he migrated to London where he successfully treated members of the aristocracy and peerage after orthodox treatment had failed to provide relief. In his work he was assisted by Dr F. W. Axham, an anaesthetist, who had been impressed by his methods. In 1911 Barker was sued for £5,000 by

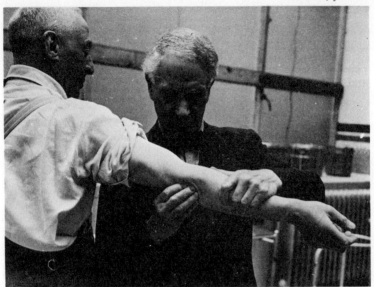

Sir Herbert Barker

the parents of a patient, who failed to respond. Whitehead testified on his behalf, as did other medical men, but the jury found for the plaintiff, to whom they awarded 20 guineas, which was virtually a victory for Barker. His costs, however, came to £3,000 but the amount of publicity the case brought was worth ten times that sum and patients flocked to him. Axham was struck off the Register by the GMC however and his career ruined.

During the 1914 war Barker performed thousands of manipulative operations on war victims, without charge, and his reputation was so great that King George V was pressed to award him a knighthood, which he did in 1922. This made no difference to the GMC, for Axham was never reinstated.

During his career Barker performed more than 40,000 manipulative operations and in 1937 was invited to lecture, demonstrate and teach his methods to students at St Thomas's Hospital, London, where they were recorded on film. Barker also believed in the natural way to health, was a vegetarian, and often indulged in short fasts of from one to three days.

Barker, J. Ellis (1870-1950). Son of a well-known medical man who studied medicine, then realised the futility of orthodox methods and turned to *homeopathy*. One of his first cases was a man who, after being under observation for four days at the Swansea General Hospital, was told he suffered from an inoperable cancer of the bowel and had only a week to live. His wife appealed to Barker for help; he was cured and in gratitude sent his benefactor 40-50 patients. Other grateful patients sent him from 20-30 apiece and his practice expanded so rapidly that within a year or two he employed three secretaries to help him with his correspondence. He cured by natural means: homeopathic remedies, a vegetarian diet and exercise. He was not a vegetarian but insisted that when diseased all patients had to renounce meat.

The medical profession discovered bran as a cure for diverticulitis in 1973; but Barker cured dozens of cases of constipation and diverticulitis by making his patients take as many as six tablespoons of bran at each meal sixty years ago! He also cured, without recourse to the knife or drugs, patients suffering from cancer, prostrate trouble and other diseases which orthodox physicians consider it impossible to cure without surgery. His books *Heal Thyself, My Testament of Healing, Good Health and Happiness, New Lives For Old,* and *Cancer: How It Is Cured and How It Can Be Prevented* have brought hope and health to thousands who could gain no help from doctors. He claimed that if taken in hand in time, there is no incurable disease.

Barley (Hordeum pratense). A species of edible grass which has considerable nutritional value, being rich in iron and vitamin B. It has long been valued by herbalists and doctors, for it cools the body, strengthens the nerves, and barley water is invaluable in kidney and bladder troubles. Barley gruel is an ideal food for convalescents and in Eastern Europe barley bread is a staple food. Pearl barley, the kind used to make barley water, consists of 11.50% water, 8.50% protein, 1.10% fat, 77.80% carbohydrates, and 2.70% mineral matter, mainly phosphorus and potassium. A very potent wine, good for the kidneys, can also be brewed from barley. It should be used in moderation.

Bates, Dr William Horatio. One of the most eminent eye specialists of his day in New York City, who gradually grew disenchanted with orthodox medicine and began to question the methods in use. 'Why', he asked, 'if glasses are the correct procedure, must they be strenghened because the eyes under their influence have weakened?' He also questioned the prevailing Helmholtz theory founded on the premise that changes in the shape of the eye lens enables it to see at varying distances; that is, one focuses by the changing of the shape of the crystalline lens. He reasoned that if a medicine is any good the doses should be weakened as the patient improves, but this did not seem to apply in the case of defective sight. Patients were given stronger glasses. So he went to the laboratory of Columbia University where he repeated the old experiments on which ophthalmology is based and discovered, to his surprise, after analysing the eyes of 20,000 school children, that eye defects are caused by the misuse of the six intrinsic muscles of the eyes, and not the lens, and if the eyes are correctly used, refractive errors can be corrected.

He found that the main reason for eye weaknesses was strain, which actually prevented the muscles from focusing correctly, and when strain was removed the eyes focused normally. Bates studied exhaustively the action and reaction of the eye and experimented on birds, fish, animals and humans. Eventually he devised a system of exercises to strengthen eye muscles, and procedures known as palming and swinging, to relieve tension. He said: 'If my findings are not what I say, I should be exposed and the public protected. If eyes can be normalised by simple, natural methods of relaxation, it is a breach of medical ethics not to give this boon to suffering humanity.'

Though Bates met with considerable opposition in America and Britain his methods are in use in Germany where the Army, Navy and Air Force have adopted them, and some *Sehenschulen* (seeing schools) have been founded. There are Bates practitioners all over the world though officialdom everywhere is reluctant to accept his methods. See: Eyes.

Bathing. The cult of bathing in order to promote health is as old as the human race. Cold baths are taken to invigorate and hot baths to cleanse and relax. History relates that sometimes Cleopatra indulged in as many as 69 baths a day in asses' milk, and during the Roman Empire bathing was brought to an art. In Ancient Greece the bath was preceded by vigorous games and then by massage; and in Roman Britain the sexes bathed together in the nude in Bath. Then the archbishops of Bremen and Cologne forbade Sunday bathing as it kept people from church, and as an act of renunciation refrained from washing their own bodies. This edict was ignored in Britain, even when in 1450 Bishop Beckyngton threatened to excommunicate all who entered the water in a state of nudity in mixed bathing places. But when he started the rumour that mixed bathing propagated venereal disease the baths emptied as if by magic, and a shocked Venetian ambassador wrote home in 1478: 'The English have many fantastic customs, notably bathing once or twice a month.'

For 300 years the cult of dirt took over and when in the seventeenth century Lady Mary Montague was told that her hands were dirty, she exclaimed: 'My hands – you should see my feet!'

Per Hendrik Ling was the first modern European to realise the value of bathing; he built the first open-air swimming baths in 1813 and popularised bathing. Gradually the cult caught on and was accelerated by the Anglo-Indian nabobs who returned with vast fortunes from India, where they had grown accustomed to bathing twice a day. They installed baths in their mansions and started a vogue. Today most homes have a bath or a shower (many have both), and the science of *hydrotherapy* is accepted as an instrument in the curative process. See: Hydrotherapy, Water.

Baunscheidt's Cure. In the eighteen forties a mechanic named Baunscheidt sat idly at an open window in a village near Bonn, nursing a wrist swollen by rheumatism. It was a warm summer evening and a swarm of mosquitos settled on his wrist, which was bitten badly. Next day the pain in his wrist had vanished. This set him thinking and he made an instrument consisting of 30 fine needles set in a small disc. By means of a spring the needles could be plunged into the skin, after which an irritant oil was rubbed into the punctures. Baunscheidt experimented on friends and found that a pustulant rash always appeared, which dried in about a week, after which the pain disappeared. So effective was his apparatus that Dr Schaunnstein, a local physician, devised a refined model by which he cured arthritis, neuritis, bursitis and lumbago, increasing his practice and making him famous. He was denounced as a quack but this did not prevent grateful patients from recommending him to friends and relatives.

Beans. Beans fall into a group known as *pulses* which are excellent sources of energy and protein. The protein in pulses varies in nature according to their origin. They lack fat, which makes them an ideal food for all who wish to keep down their weight, but are hard to digest. Into this category fall the garden pea, haricot bean, broad bean, horse bean, chick pea, cow pea, lentils and St John's bread.

When beans are green they contain comparatively little protein (from 4.00–7.00%) but when dried this increases enormously. Beans should always be thoroughly cooked and no more than two or three ounces a day eaten. In many tropical and semi-tropical countries they serve as an adequate substitute for flesh foods. The following table gives some idea of their respective food values:

Average chemical composition per cent.

	Water	Protein	Fat	Carbo-hydrates	Minerals
Beans (dried)	14.76	24.30	1.60	49.00	3.26
Beans (blackeye)	8.48	1.28	61.28	4.78	
Chick Peas	14.80	13.00	1.60	51.50	3.76
Cow Peas (dried)	13.00	21.40	1.40	60.80	3.40
Horse Beans	14.00	18.00	0.50	50.50	2.75
Kidney Beans (dried)	13.60	23.12	2.28	53.63	3.53
Kidney Beans (green)	84.10	3.90	0.20	8.30	0.70
Lima Beans (dried)	10.40	18.10	1.50	65.90	4.10
Lima Beans (green)	74.60	7.10	0.70	22.90	1.70
Peas (dried)	15.00	22.85	1.80	52.40	2.58
Peas (green)	74.60	7.00	0.50	16.90	1.00
St. John's Bread	17.30	5.70	1.10	67.00	2.50
Soya Beans	10.75	34.00	16.80	33.70	4.75
String Beans (fresh)	84.10	3.90	0.20	8.30	1.20

The composition of mineral matter is one in every 1,000 parts of water free substance.

Beer. Many people believe, mistakenly, that they can live almost exclusively on beers, of which there are many varieties ranging from pale ale to stout. Beer does not remain in the stomach any longer than water and leaves it completely in about 1½ hours. As beers contain digestible carbohydrates they must be rated as foods, but one pint of good ale contains as many carbohydrates as one and one fifth ounces of bread. A pint of ale contains 310 calories, strong ale 428, and stout 282; and a glass of milk (about half a pint) 184. This does not mean that beers are as good a source of energy as milk or that they are as good foods, for they are deficient in calcium, iron, phosphorus and most of the vitamins, except B.

If taken with meals beers delay the chemical processes of digestion, though *one* glass of good beer may aid digestion by increasing appetite and producing more gastric juice. Beers and stouts are mild soporifics and any benefits they have may be largely psychological. Taken in moderation – a pint or even two a day – they can be beneficial, but in excess of that they tend to fatten. Good beer is difficult to find for most of the commercial products contain chemical additives to produce fizz and froth. The best beer is home-brewed.

Bee Stings. For centuries countrymen have believed that bee stings were a sovereign cure for rheumatism, arthritis, lumbago and gout and Charles the Great and Ivan the Terrible of Russia were cured of gout by bee stings. Bee venom has been analysed and found to contain formic acid, histamine and phosphate of magnesium. Dr H. Garin, the South African scientist and apiarist, says that bee venom is closely related to the poison of the mamba, the deadliest African reptile. 'It is now known,' he said, 'that the bee's poison is a very complex body. The active part appears to be a lecithid, a substance more or less related to the active part of snake venom, and some special mysterious alkaloid substance related to the very active poisons like strychnine or belladonna.'

In Russia sensational claims for bee venom have been made in cases of neuritis, neuralgia, malaria, exophthalmic goitre and some skin and eye diseases, and in his book *Curative Properties of Honey and Bee Venom* the scientist N. Yourish gives case histories of patients successfully treated by bee venom. Scientists from Guy's Hospital, the Kennedy Institute of Rheumatology, and University College, London, have extracted a substance from bee venom called Peptide 401 which is 100 times as powerful as cortisone in the treatment of rheumatism, though it is extremely costly and five pounds of venom produces only an insignificant amount. Still the cheapest and most effective method is to be stung by a bee.

A Mrs Julia Owen of Bromley, Kent, who keeps 10,000,000 bees, runs a bee-sting clinic where bees held by tweezers, are applied to patients' necks, and some of them are stung as many as 50 times. She has some remarkable cures to her credit, claiming successes with well known patients such as Norman Dodds MP, whose arthritis was cured, and Robert Helpman, whose career as a ballet dancer was threatened by arthritis in the knees. 'Now,' he says, 'I can dance for hours and hours and never feel an ache.' Hundreds of lesser known people have also been cured after being stung by bees.

Berries. Berries are not usually considered an essential part of the human diet, but into this category fall a number of many-seeded pulpy fruits, including the tomato, which are used to provide flavour and nutrition. Their value lies mainly in their flavour, the fruit sugar they contain, pure water content, and vitamins. When refined sugar is eaten body cells are rapidly broken down to furnish the blood with the necessary alkaline elements to neutralise the carbonic acid resulting from the oxidation of carbon. Fruit sugar is intimately associated with alkaline elements while refined sugar is deficient in organic salts and cannot, except for a very brief period, maintain the life processes of the body. Berries help to keep the blood in balance and the body in health.

Blackberry. The most common of all English berries found in hedgerows in every part of Britain. May be eaten raw or cooked. Contain 84.00% water, 0.40% protein, 0.50% fat, 13.00% carbohydrates, and 0.50% mineral salts, mainly potassium, calcium and phosphorus; and vitamin C.

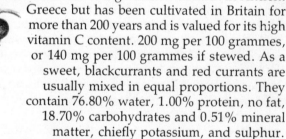

Blackcurrant. Believed to have originated in Corinth in Ancient Greece but has been cultivated in Britain for more than 200 years and is valued for its high vitamin C content. 200 mg per 100 grammes, or 140 mg per 100 grammes if stewed. As a sweet, blackcurrants and red currants are usually mixed in equal proportions. They contain 76.80% water, 1.00% protein, no fat, 18.70% carbohydrates and 0.51% mineral matter, chiefly potassium, and sulphur.

Boysenberry. A man-made hybrid having the loganberry and raspberry as parents, and named after Rudolph Boysen of California who, after innumerable crossings produced the species. It is virtually seedless, has a very small core, is over two inches long and produces 25% more juice than any other

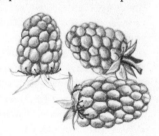

23

bramble plant, and far more vitamin C; as much, in fact, as orange juice. There are about 50 berries to a quart and an acre will grow 435 plants yielding six tons of berries (about 7,000 quarts). It should be better known as it flourishes on poor soil.

Elderberry. One of the least appreciated but one of the most valuable of all berries. Every part of the elder tree has medicinal

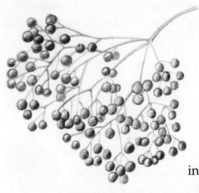

uses: root, stem, leaves and berries. The berries are diaphoretic, emmolient, alterative and diuretic. An infusion of the flowers with peppermint and yarrow is good for colds. Warm elderflower water soothes the eyes and hot elderberry wine is widely used as part of the treatment for colds and influenza. A very pleasant cure, for if made properly elderberry wine has the bouquet and flavour of vintage port. The berries can also be made into a tasty jam.

The juice of the berries mixed with a little honey is an excellent specific for laryngitis, pharyngitis, stomatitis, Vincent's angina, sciatica and rheumatism. Elderberries are rich in vitamin C but unfortunately no analysis seems to have been made of them.

Gooseberry. One of the more acid berries, to be eaten only when fully ripe. Usually made into jam with apple; into pies and tarts, or stewed and eaten with cream or custard. Traditionally eaten as a blood purifier in spring. Contains 85.70% water, 0.50% protein, no fat, 8.40% carbohydrates, and 0.40% mineral matter, mainly potassium, phosphorus and calcium. A much under-rated fruit. Gather when fully ripe, hold a berry in one hand and pierce the other end with a pointed knife; then squeeze the pulp into a dish. This can be done easily and a fair sized bowl filled rapidly. Mix with a little honey, top with cream and you have a dish fit for a king.

When making jam, throw a head of elderflowers into the pan. When the flowers pass into the jam, remove the stalk. The flowers give it a superb aroma and a flavour like that of muscatels.

Grape. Few consider the grape to be a berry but it falls into that category and nutritionally is the most valuable of them all. The flavour of the grape depends on the soil in which it is grown. Many years ago Lahmann advocated the 'Grape Cure' in Germany and since then naturopaths have found it invaluable in the treatment of many diseases.

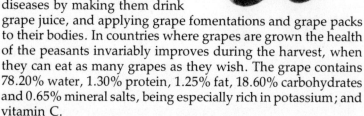

Sophocles and Hippocrates wrote that invalids were cured by the juice of the grape, and Celsus, Plinius and Galen advocated the eating of grapes for health. Shackleton devised a grape cure for cancer, and Edgar Cayce cured patients of many diseases by making them drink grape juice, and applying grape fomentations and grape packs to their bodies. In countries where grapes are grown the health of the peasants invariably improves during the harvest, when they can eat as many grapes as they wish. The grape contains 78.20% water, 1.30% protein, 1.25% fat, 18.60% carbohydrates and 0.65% mineral salts, being especially rich in potassium; and vitamin C.

Loganberry. Produced originally by Judge Logan, who crossed blackberries with raspberries. The loganberry is larger than either, possesses the qualities of both but has a mellower flavour and contains vitamin C. Eventually it will probably be ousted by the Boysenberry.

Mulberry. Once flourished in every English garden but today is a comparative rarity. It is like a large blackberry with the pointed shape of a loganberry. Some are inches long. It can be eaten as dessert, made into jam or wine, or used for tarts and pies. It consists of 84.70% water, 0.40% protein, no fat, 14.30% carbohydrates, and 0.60% mineral matter.

Raspberry. A delicious berry with a sub-acid or rasping flavour. Usually eaten with cream or made into jam, or used as a filling for pies and tarts. Contains numerous little pips which are so sharp that they are apt to lodge

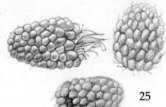

25

under dental plates and are avoided by those who wear them. Contains 85.80% water, 1.00% protein, no fat, 9.70% carbohydrates, and 0.60% mineral matter, mainly potassium, sulphur and phosphorus.

Red Currant. Usually made into jam, and mixed with blackcurrants into a sweet, or as a filling for tarts and pies. Contains 82.20% water, 0.30% protein, no fat, 11.30% carbohydrates, and 0.45% mineral matter, mainly potassium and sulphur.

Strawberry. Most popular of all English berries and considered a delicacy to be eaten with cream. A good blood cleanser which

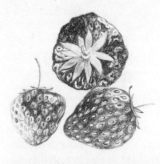

Linnaeus, the Father of Botany, ate in large quantities to cure his gout. Too many strawberries, however, tend to produce gall stones. Weight for weight the strawberry has as much vitamin C as the *orange*. It consists of 87.70% water, 1.00% protein, 0.60% fat, 7.70% carbohydrates, and 0.80% mineral matter, mainly sodium, potassium, calcium, phosphorus and silicon.

Bircher-Benner, Dr Max, MD. An early pioneer of food science and a vegetarian, who felt that the medical profession paid too

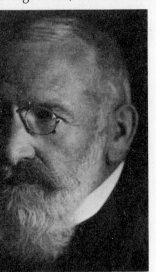

Dr Max Bircher-Benner

much attention to signs and symptoms of disease and not enough to its cause. In 1897 he founded the Bircher-Benner Clinic in Zurich, which is known throughout the world as a Nature Cure Centre. 'Incurables' from every continent flocked to him and he either cured or greatly relieved them. After numerous experiments he devised a 'perfect' food which he called muesli, containing all the constituents needed for health and growth. When given to convalescing patients it was found that most of them gained strength and vigour from the first day. Into a bowl he mixed one tablespoon of honey; two tablespoons of cream; two tablespoons of hot water; one tablespoon of oatmeal; the juice of half a lemon; two medium size apples, grated; and one tablespoon of hazel nuts. It was always served fresh and fed to patients twice a day; and nothing else.

He was one of the first to advocate the treatment of tuberculosis by means of fresh air, sunlight and diet and during his lifetime had thousands of disciples. He also placed food into a number of categories; into the first class he put natural, fresh uncooked orchard fruits, berries, nuts almonds, vegetable fruits, leaves, stems, roots or bulbs, and seeds; into the second those foods subjected to heat; and in the third all animal tissues, which he said were the chief sources of arthritis. Although he was substantially correct, discoveries in the field of vitamins, etc., have caused food reformers to modify some of his theories.

Blistering. The skin is a major organ through which noxious elements in the body are eliminated. For centuries physicians have applied blistering salves, plasters behind the ears, on the shaved head and on the back of the neck to relieve deafness, catarrh, gout, constipation and nervous complaints. Today many practitioners of fringe medicine use blistering, with considerable success.

Blood. The blood is a fluid organ which has many functions: (1) it carries oxygen to the tissues (2) carbon dioxide from the tissues to the lungs where it is expelled (3) white cells to the tissues of infection (4) waste products to the kidneys (5) sugar to the liver where it is stored as glycogen (6) in disease it carries away bacteria and blood clots (7) it is invaluable in nutrition, respiration and excretion (8) maintains the acid-base balance of the body and its water balance (9) helps to regulate body temperature, for blood consists mainly of water which has a high specific heat, and it travels at such a speed that it can transfer large amounts of heat from one area to another and so enables the body to maintain a constant temperature despite changes outside it.

Blood-Letting See: Venesection.

Bone. Bone is not solid, as many people imagine. There are two kinds: (1) spongy (2) compact. Spongy bone lies inside and is protected from injury by compact bone. Bone consists of thousands of tiny blood vessels and active cells called *osteoblasts* which create new bone, and other cells called *osteoclasts* which tear down old bone and pass it into the blood from which it is excreted.

Weight for weight bone is stronger than mild steel but unlike steel, bone has two kinds of strength: it resists compression or crushing forces; it resists tensile or disrupting forces; and in these respects bone is superior to cast iron, wrought iron and wood. Experiments on the femurs of rats show that the average breaking stress to bending is 35,000 lb per square inch compared with 40,000 for cast iron; but bone is flexible and one third as heavy as cast iron. It is also three times as strong as most timber and half as strong again as mild steel, both of which are much heavier. If the axial load is increased five times by jumping from a height, the strength of bone is shown to be 140 times greater than necessary. Bones are not merely props; they have a 'give' about them which wood and steel lack and, 'The strength of bone,' says J. C. Koch, 'may be compared with that of reinforced concrete.'* In order that bones should be strong and healthy, minerals and vitamins are necessary; of the minerals calcium, magnesium and phosphorus are the most important, and of the vitamins, A, C and D.

Bonemeal. The bones of healthy, selected cattle, ground as fine as flour and taken with water or milk, or in soups. Dr S. G. Harootian, visiting oral surgeon to the Worcester City Hospital, Worcester, Mass., USA, and Dr Elizabeth B. Martin, MD, of Oshawa, Ontario, carried out separately and unknown to each other, experiments with bone meal. Harootian gave bone meal to patients suffering from psychological torpor and *caries*, and achieved dramatic results. Dr Martin fed bonemeal to children with dental troubles, and to pregnant women, and achieved equally gratifying results, with no side effects. Bonemeal therapy is gradually gaining adherents.

Dr William N. Macartney, MD, says in *Fifty Years A Country Doctor* that bonemeal contains all the minerals of natural bone, in exactly the correct proportions and bonemeal tablets can be given safely. 'In certain conditions it is as nearly a specific cure as anything we are likely to meet in this vale of tears.'

Bradbury, Parnell. A gifted writer, it was however, as an osteopath and chiropractor in Sussex that Parnell Bradbury is best known, and all interested in health and particularly the spine, should read *Healing by Hand*, *The Mechanics of Healing*, and

*Laws of Bone Architecture: J. C. Koch

Adventures In Healing, which give laymen an insight into these arts.

His outlook was broad; he was interested in fundamentals and in healing the body as a whole. He was a *food reformer* and did not hesitate to recommend homeopathic remedies where he felt these would help his patients for he realised that no single system of therapy had all the answers for the sick. He became interested in *Psionic Medicine,* a way of healing which involves intuition and the sensitivity

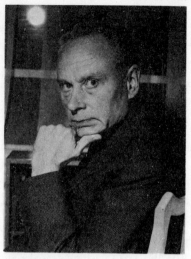

Parnell Bradbury

of the practitioner. Like all good healers, he was not concerned as much with symptoms as with underlying causes; and when these have been eliminated the self-healing mechanisms of the body take over and restore health.

Bran. After the protective outer husk has been removed the wheat grain is covered by bran, which comprises 13.5% of the berry. It consists of 12.40% water, 16.6% protein, 3.50% fat, 63.10% carbohydrates and 4.80% mineral matter, mainly phosphorus, potassium and magnesium. For nearly a century vegetarians and food reformers have stated that flour containing the entire wheat berry was essential for health, though they did not know why, as vitamins were unknown and the mineral content of wheat had not been analysed. The medical profession scorned their claims and remained sceptical.

Ellis Barker, Allinson, MacCarrison, Wrench, Austin, Aykroyd and others, lauded the virtues of wholewheat flour products which contained bran, but it was not till 1974 that the medical profession at large acknowledged that bran played a valuable part in nutrition and was a cure for *diverticulitis* – just plain bran such as is fed to horses, and not the packed stuff mixed with sugar and processed.

Brazil Nut. Fruit of the brazil tree, a native of Brazil, which attains a height of 150 feet, with no branches for the first 40 or 50 feet. It grows a foot in the first year, 20 in the next four, and produces

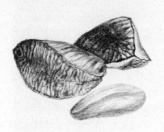

nuts in about nine years. From 12 to 25 nuts are encased in a hard shell weighing from two to four pounds, and a full grown tree will produce about 300 nuts, or 1,000 lb of brazils. The nut contains 4.10% water, 17.40% protein, 65.00% fat, 5.70% carbohydrates and 3.30% mineral matter, mainly phosphorus, potassium and calcium.

Bread, White. It is now accepted by nutritionists that white flour products contribute to many modern diseases such as constipation, rhuematism, arthritis, dental caries, diabetes and obesity. White flour contains 12.60% water, 10.20% protein, 0.90% fat, 74.70% carbohydrates, 0.50% mineral matter; a very poor source of minerals.

Bread, Wholewheat. As foods, wholewheat products are far superior to those made from refined flour; even enriched white bread to which *synthetic vitamins* have been added. Wholewheat flour contains *bran,* which has been extracted from all refined flours, and is far richer in vitamin A, B_1, B_2, niacin, and the richest source of vitamin E in most diets. White flour contains no vitamin E. Unfortunately the public as a whole continues to ignore wholewheat bread and the government does nothing to educate it. Wholewheat flour contains 13.40% water, 13.60% protein, 1.90% fat, 69.10% carbohydrates, and 2.00% mineral matter, mainly phosphorus, potassium and magnesium.

Breathing. If respiration ceased in the normal man or woman for more than four minutes, death would result, though in a few instances people are known to have survived after five minutes. The purpose of breathing is to inhale air, which consists of two colourless, odourless gases: nitrogen 79% and oxygen 21% – and other gases.

For metabolism to continue, complex chemical substances must be broken down (katabolism) and body tissues created from simple substances (anabolism). For these functions the body must be provided with air, water, food, sunshine and light. During respiration waste products are eliminated through lungs, mouth, kidneys, bowels and skin in the form of solids, liquids and gases.

During inhalation the blood takes up oxygen, which changes in colour from blue to bright red. Oxygenated blood is carried by the arteries to every part of the body and the venous system returns the blood to the heart with its load of carbon dioxide, a poisonous gas, which is carried in the blood in the form of sodium bicarbonate, which is necessary for the functioning of the heart. Carbon dioxide is expelled during exhalation.

Brewer's Yeast. Yeast is a fungus which if fed on sugar multiplies in volume many millions of times within hours. It is used to make bread rise and the liquor in barley ferment, transforming it into beer. At the turn of the century Max Fleischmann, a Hungarian refugee in America, succeeded in producing dried yeast in a test tube of yeast plants and by selling his product became a millionaire. Later cultures of yeast known as *Tortula utilis* were cultivated from the atmosphere by using ammonia, and in 1941 a committee was set up in Jamaica under Professor Raistrick to produce yeast for human food.

It is now known that yeast is a high quality protein essential for growth, and a prime source of nicotinic acid or niacin, used in the prevention and cure of beri-beri and pellagra. The protein in Brewer's Yeast is 50% of its dry weight and each gramme contains 2.10 mg of *aneurin*, 5 mg of *riboflavin*, and 40–45 mg of nicotinic acid. From one eighth to half an ounce a day, if added to foods one normally eats, will supply all the protein needed. It was found that children given eight grammes of dried yeast in biscuit form for five days a week, in addition to their usual diet, increased much faster in weight than children who did not receive this ration.

Bronchitis. Derived from the Greek *brogkhos*, windpipe, and *itis*, a suffix used to denote inflammation. It is 'inflammation of the mucous membrane of the windpipe'. The disease usually starts with an ordinary cold which extends to the larynx, causing huskiness of speech and pain on swallowing. The windpipe become raw and dry and a painful cough results. The patient feels ill, heavy, tired, has pains in the back and the joints ache. There is tightness in the upper portion of the chest and the temperature rises. Orthodox methods alleviate but seldom cure. Naturopaths advocate short fasts followed by a reform of the diet to restore the balance of the blood, breathing exercises and, where possible, a removal of the patient to a part of the country where the air is free from coal dust and industrial gases. Osteopathy and hot and cold packs will accelerate the cure.

Buckwheat. Recently introduced into Britain but popular in America, Brittany and Holland, where it has been eaten for centuries in the form of porridge and fritters. It contains 13.27% water, 11.41% protein, 2.68% fat, 68.79% carbohydrates, and 2.38% mineral matter, mainly phosphorus, potassium and magnesium. See: Rutin.

Butter. From ancient times considered a valuable food. It is the most easily digestible of fats and an excellent source of vitamin A. The colour of butter varies according to the region in which cows are fed: Channel Island butter is almost marigold in colour; Ayrshire butter is much paler; so manufacturers often add a soluble yellow dye to pale butters. Butter contains a high degree of cholesterol, which has been blamed for the increasing incidence of heart disease, but Professor Yudkin and other authorities state that there is no direct evidence for the theory connecting butter fat with coronary thrombosis and that other factors must be taken into account, such as the wrong diet, stress and lack of exercise. Cow's butter contains 11.00% water, 1.00% protein, 85.00% fat, no carbohydrates, and 3.00% mineral matter, mainly sodium, sulphur and chlorine. It also contains more vitamin D than any foods except fish oils.

Butter is not essential for health and *vegans* do not touch it, mainly because of the cruelty involved in the rearing of animals for slaughter.

C

C-Vitamin. See: Vitamin C.

Caffeine. A stimulant drug found in tea, coffee and cocoa, which affects the nervous system and the kidneys. Caffeine inhibits the digestion of boiled starch to maltose by the ptyalin in the saliva but the effect is almost negligible unless the beverage is very strong or the digestion weak. The amount of caffeine in tea and coffee does not differ appreciably if both are infused for five minutes or less.

Calcium. An element that enters into the composition of bones and teeth as phosphate and carbonate. It is absorbed probably in inorganic form in the small intestine and this absorption is aided by the presence of vitamin D. A lack of calcium leads to osteoporosis of the bones and a lack of vitamin D to rickets and osteomalacia.

Canned Foods. Fruit and vegetables freshly picked and eaten are, if grown in composted soil, superior in taste and nutritive value to canned goods, but as much of the food in shops and markets is neither fresh nor grown in compost, a great deal of canned food, which is canned very soon after picking, may be as good or even better. Modern canning methods are so efficient that in glass containers 70–75% of the vitamin C is conserved; and in cans 80–86%, and very little vitamin A is lost.

Carbohydrates. Compounds of hydrogen and carbon in the proportion of 2:1, and water. As they contain water and the Greek word for water is *hudor,* they derive their name from a combination of all three words.

Carbohydrates are found mainly in all fruit and vegetable tissue and form a very large proportion of our diet. The most important are sugars glucose, fructose and lactose, and cellulose; and in the human body, glycogen and glucose. Cellulose is the material which makes up cell walls and the woody fibres of plants. Its indigestible bulk is necessary for the movements of the alimentary canal. Carbohydrates are converted into fat and provide the body with energy.

It is virtually impossible to live on a diet devoid of all carbohydrates and slimmers who attempt to exist on proteins alone under the impression that carbohydrates are fattening, defeat themselves because the liver converts the amino-acids in proteins and metabolises them into glucose and fatty acids, and turns the amino group into urea, thus rendering those amino-acids useless for tissue building. As far as proteins are concerned, the slimmer might just as well be starving. Carbohydrates are essential not only for health, but for life itself. See: Hay diet, Proteins, Fats.

Caries, Dental. A disease of the the teeth caused by the state of the saliva, which erodes the enamel, eventually exposes the nerve and causes agony. It has been proved that if wholewheat products are substituted for white; and honey and molasses for white sugar; and fresh fruit and vegetables grown in compost are eaten; and milk, eggs and fish oils added to the diet, the teeth will be free from caries. It is one of the most common diseases in Britain, America, Australia and New Zealand but is rare in countries where a 'civilised' diet is unknown.

Carrot. A root vegetable outstanding for its high vitamin A content: 6,700 IU per 100 grammes. Dr E. L. Severingham, Medical Consultant to the Vitamin Information Bureau, USA, says that cooking releases a substance from which the body manufactures vitamin A more easily. A small carrot eaten raw after a meal

cleanses the enamel and helps to prevent caries. The carrot
contains 87.00% water, 1.00% protein, 0.20% fat, 9.40% carbohydrates, and 0.90% mineral salts, mainly potassium, sodium and phosphorus.

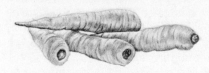

Castor Oil. Children, except in remote country districts, are no longer dosed with castor oil. This oil is, however, extremely valuable in the treatment of severe cuts. It is a gipsy remedy and sometimes used by farmers who believe in the old methods. Crude castor oil and not the refined kind should be applied to wounds of both animals and humans. It cleans and cures rapidly and effectively. This simple cure has been neglected since the advent of antibiotics, but castor oil heals without any side effects.

Cellulose. Indigestible fibre contained in vegetables, known as 'roughage' which, though having no known nutritional value, is essential to the peristaltic action of the bowel. The rate of passage of foods through the large intestine is increased by vegetable foods, either because of mechanical stimulus due to coarse indigestible fibres or by the chemical breakdown products of vegetable cell walls.

Cheese. Cheese is a valuable food, especially for lacto-vegetarians and there are an infinite variety of cheeses available in Britain. Major Rance, the owner of Wells of Streatley-on-Thames, sells more than 150 varieties made from the milk of cows, ewes and goats. Because most cheeses contain a high proportion of fat they are not easily digested and so should be well masticated. Grated cheese is more easily digested than if not grated. Nearly 90% of cheese protein is retained in the body and 90% of its energy is available. Four ounces of cheese, 8 oz of wholewheat bread and 2 oz of watercress form an almost nutritionally complete meal and contain about 1,000 calories. Cheeses vary in their food value but a good average hard cheese contains 38.80% water, 23.75% protein, 30.00% fat, 1.50% carbohydrates and 4.50% mineral matter, mainly sodium, calcium and phosphorus. Cheese is an excellent food because a wide range of dishes can be made with it.

Chemicals In Food. It is estimated that more than 2,500 chemicals are added to foods in order to preserve, dye and flavour them. Many such agents advertised as 'safe' have later been proved to be harmful and capable of causing diseases such as tumours and cancer. In 1976, for instance, the National Politechnical Institute, USA, stated that almost all food produced in Mexico was contaminated with cancer-causing agents containing Aldrin, banned by other nations. In Britain nearly 30 substances are used for flavouring, more than 30 for preserving, at least six for anti-caking, twelve or more for stabilising, more than 30 as sequestrants, about ten as emulsifying agents, about 80 as miscellaneous additives, and hundreds for all sorts of reasons. Some, such as *agar-agar* and accacia (gum arabic), which are used as stabilisers, are harmless but many of the others accumulate in the system for years and cause degenerative diseases.

Cherry. A delicious but under-valued fruit which until recently has been ignored by dieticians. In 1972 Dr Ludwig Blau, Ph.D., who suffered severely from gout, wheeled his chair to the fridge and ignoring all advice, consumed an entire bowl of cherries. Next morning the pain in his big toe had vanished. He experimented and soon had twelve case histories of patients 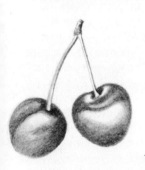 with either gout or arthritis who after eating cherries or drinking cherry wine, were relieved from pain. Cherries do not hasten the excretion of uric acid which is said to cause the disease; they merely prevent its crystallisation. Apparently all varieties of cherries are equally effective, eaten fresh or canned. Acid cherries are a good source of vitamin A, and both sweet and acid contain vitamin C and traces of thiamine, *riboflavin* and niacin. Dr J. Walters, who specialises in nutrition and dermatology, says that cherries give added vitality, help to digest and assimilate food and remove the products of congestion. The cherry contains 79.80% water, 1.00% protein, 0.80% fat, 16.70% carbohydrates, and 0.70% mineral matter, being specially rich in potassium and phosphorus.

Chestnut. In Britain chestnuts are rarely eaten as a vegetable but they appear during Christmas as stuffing for geese and turkeys, and are roasted in front of an open fire after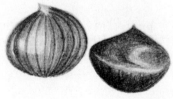

35

dinner. Vegetarians use them, however, in a variety of dishes and nut-meats. Dried chestnuts contain 5.90% water, 10.70% protein, 7.00% fat, 74.20% carbohydrates and 2.20% mineral matter, mainly potassium.

Chiropractic. A system founded by *D. D. Palmer,* who realised that disease is the result of certain alterations in the body to which it cannot adapt itself, and that these disturbed conditions can be remedied by thrusts and pressures of the human hand on sections of the spine. Most structural deviations are sublaxations of a vertebra – a fixation of a spinal bone within its normal range of movement, causing nerve irritation. When thrusts are applied these displacements are corrected and health restored. The name 'chiropractic' was coined by the Rev. Samuel Weed from the Greek *chiro,* hand, and *praktikos,* 'done by hand.' See: Palmer. In America the chiropractor is known as a chiropratic physician and the equal of an M.D. He can diagnose, prescribe drugs, perform surgery and practise psychiatry.

Chlorine. The body of a man 15$\bar{0}$ lb in weight contains 105 grammes of chlorine, which exists almost entirely as a soluble chloride and mainly as common salt (sodium chloride). It assists in the formation of digestive juices, principally the gastric juices. The mineral matter of blood serum consists largely of sodium chloride, which favours and sustains the generation and conductance of electric currents.

Cholesterol. Saturated fats; that is, the solid ones such as the fats from meats – lard, dripping and butter – are supposed to raise blood cholesterol levels, a theory which has never been satisfactorily proved. There is no evidence that these fats and dairy products alone are conducive to heart disease, there being other factors as well to account for the accumulation of cholesterol in the arteries. See: Butter, Fat.

Christian Science. Religion founded by *Mary Baker Eddy* which has some 350 churches in Britain and followers in every continent. The religion is a conventional Protestant one, which forbids smoking and alcoholic liquors, drugs, and even discussion of physical ailments because 'sick thoughts make sick bodies'. All disease, they say, originates in the mind and is usually the product of fear. It is permissible, however, to summon help for broken bones and contagious diseases, and decayed teeth may be extracted. Some astonishing cures have been recorded, including such diseases as cancer; for the mind cures all. See: Eddy, Mary Baker.

Chromotherapy. When 'white' light such as sunlight, passes through a prism, it is split into seven colours: violet, indigo, blue, green, yellow, orange and red. Chromotherapy is based on the theory that every colour has a vibration-rate different from that of other colours. These are ether-vibrations and differ from sound-vibrations for they are much smaller and vibrate at a far greater rate. Red light rays, for instance, are 1/300,000 th of an inch and violet rays 1/600,000th.

Colours are divided into groups: warm and cold; stimulating and tranquillising; those that are complementary and those that are not, etc. There are altogether more than 100,000 colours and shades though the average person can detect no more than about 150.

Healing by colour has been practised for thousands of years, by the Hindus, Tibetans, Chinese, Navajo Indians, Greeks and Egyptians; in Ancient Ireland and by the Early Christian Church. Only recently, however, have scientists paid serious thought to this type of therapy and today a school of colour healers has emerged which uses colour allied to music to cure a multitude of diseases, especially those of the mind, which resist orthodox forms of healing.

Cider. The word cider is derived from the Hebrew *Shekar* (through the Greek *sikera*) meaning strong drink generally, and applied to apple wine, for cider is a true wine if one accepts as a general definition the result of fermenting fruit juice and that alone. Cider orchards are confined to a few areas in France, England, Germany, Spain, Switzerland and northern states of America. Experts say that English cider is the best of all. Although regarded by some as almost a temperance drink, cider has an alcoholic content greater than that of beer and 'hard cider' or applejack can put those unaccustomed to it, under the table. Pure cider is regarded by many as a cure for rheumatism and taken in moderate quantities is a health drink.

Citrus Fruit. *Lemons, limes,* grapefruit, *oranges,* tangerines and pumelos come into this category as all of them contain ascorbic acid (citric acid) and malonic acids which counteract and cure scurvy and other skin diseases. Diluted with water the juice of these fruits is of great value during fasting.

Cocoa. The cocoa bean is the fruit of *Theobroma cacao* and was introduced into Europe from Mexico by the Spaniards. Though known as a beverage before tea or coffee it has never attained the popularity of either. Cocoa is produced when the bean is pulped, roasted and ground, and the powder can be drunk when mixed with milk and sugar, or eaten in slab form, as chocolate. Cocoa is a mild stimulant containing caffeine, tannin and oxalic acid. Cocoa contains 6.30% water, 21.50% protein, 27.30% fat, 31.60% carbohydrates and 5.20% mineral matter, mainly potassium and phosphorus. Chocolate contains 58.50% carbohydrates and is not advocated for slimmers, but is a good, convenient food for all who indulge in hard physical exercise. As the fat is not easily digested the young and vigorous can eat far more chocolate than the elderly and old.

Cod Liver Oil. Valuable for the formation of bones and teeth and for the health of eyes. A rich source of vitamin A and D; also contains some E and K. Used in the treatment of rickets but the taste of the oil is so unpleasant that it is best given to children in tablet form.

Coffee. The coffee bean is the fruit of *Coffaea arabica*, grown originally in Arabia. When roasted, ground into powder and infused in boiling water it makes a pleasant, stimulating beverage, taken without or with milk and sugar. The secret of good coffee is to make it fresh, strong and hot, in which case a cupful will contain 1.7 grains of *caffeine* and 3.24 grains of tannin; about the same amount of both as in a cup of tea. It is a stimulant, affecting the nervous system, and a diuretic, affecting the kidneys. It clears the mind, abolishes a sense of fatigue and in many people, induces sleeplessness. *Dr Bernard Aschner* says that small amounts of coffee if taken after breakfast or lunch are harmless, and indeed, may be beneficial. 'This excellent means of quickly restoring a flabby or hyperacid stomach will harm no heart.' 'The best way to drink it is fresh, strong and black. Do not drink coffee that has been standing for hours because it then turns into a substance noxious to the stomach. See: Caffeine, Tannin.

Cola Drinks. Cola drinks are bad for health, especially if taken regularly, as they are by children. They are rich in *glucose* and refined *sugar*, both of which are harmful to the health and teeth. Long after the cola has disappeared down one's throat the sugar remains in the mouth and coats the teeth, eating away the enamal. See: Glucose.

Cold. See: Temperature.

Cold Baths. See: Hydrotherapy, Bathing.

Cold Water Cure. See: Hydrotherapy.

Comfrey (Symphitum officinalis). Also called knit-bone, and known to the Crusaders for repairing bones. No known herb or medicine helps to repair bones so speedily. Its mucilaginous properties come from the alkaloid *Allantoin,* which encourages cell proliferation. About 70 years ago Charles MacAlister, MD, FRCP, Consultant Physician to Liverpool Hospitals, successfully used comfrey for fractures and superficial ulcers. His treatment is described in *Comfrey, An Ancient Medicinal Remedy.* It can be used externally as a poultice or an ointment, and internally as an infusion or taken in tablet form. It can be grown in any garden, is one of the richest sources of Vitamin B_{12} and can be eaten cooked, in stews, or fresh in salads.

Compost. See: Humus.

Constipation. A disease which is the cause of many other diseases, but which can be cured by a diet in which salads and fruit, and 100% *wholewheat bread* and *bran* play a considerable part. Dried and fresh *figs* and beetroot are excellent foods for moving the bowels. Constipation often results in *diverticulitis.* See: Purgatives.

Copper. The body of a 150 lb man contains about 51 grains of copper, which is found in the lungs, liver and heart, with traces in other organs. It is generally thought that a deficiency of iron is the prime cause of anaemia; but anaemia has been present when iron salts were abundant, but copper absent. The catalytic action of copper helps to transfer iron from food to the blood. Copper is found in liver, wheat germ, oats, rye, corn, barley, nuts, legumes, dried fruits, fresh fruits, leafy vegetables, poultry and fish. Acid foods should not be cooked in copper pans unless they are lined with tin as the amount of copper eaten away and deposited in food can be poisonous.

Corn. The seed of all cereal or farinacious plants; thus in England corn is wheat or barley; in Scotland oats; in America corn on the cob etc.

Coué, Emil (1857-1926). Psychotherapist born in Troyes, France. Studied the technique and uses of hypnosis under H. Bernheim and A. A. Liebault and made patients repeat daily: 'Every day and in every way I am becoming better and better.' This therapy, called auto-suggestion, based on imagination, was a form of self-hypnosis. Constant repetition of the sentence made the idea sink into the subconscious, eliminating thoughts that caused disease and distress. Coue', who had a world following, stressed that he was not a healer but taught people to heal themselves. He claimed that suggestion effected organic changes and during his lifetime had an immense following in France, USA and Britain.

Cucumber. For centuries the cucumber has been recommended
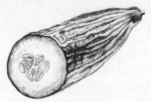
by herbalists for its internal and external cleansing properties and for clearing the skin of blemishes. Not till recently, however, has it been analysed and the high opinion held of it has been confirmed. It contains 95.60% water, 1.20% protein, 0.10% fat, 2.30% carbohydrates, and 0.44% mineral matter, being rich in potassium and having a fair proportion of phosphorus, chlorine, calcium and sulphur.

D

D Vitamin. See: Vitamin D.

Dandelion. *(Taraxacum officinalis)*. Every part of the dandelion has some medicinal value. The root dried, and ground, is made into a 'coffee', and is a mild laxative. Part of the root under the bark, will if taken regularly, cure the most stubborn constipation. The leaves, which contain ten times as much *vitamin C* as *oranges*, are slightly bitter and add piquancy to salads or sandwiches. Every part of the dandelion helps to purify the blood, is antacid, and will assist in curing anaemia, dropsy, debility, heart weakness, high blood pressure, liver, kidney and gall bladder troubles, piles, rheumatism and skin disorders. Gipsies, who use a number of herbs, rely mainly on the dandelion and *nettle* for curing most ills. Jack Boyce, whose family have been seedsmen for more than 100 years, claims that the regular eating of dandelion leaves makes for longevity. An excellent, slightly bitter, tonic wine can be made from dandelion flowers. The dandelion contains 85.50% water, 2.80% protein, 0.70% fat, 7.45% carbohydrates and 1.90% mineral salts, being very rich in potassium and containing significant quantities of calcium, sodium, magnesium, phosphorus and silicon.

Date. Probably the oldest cultivated fruit, as date palms were grown for food more than 6,000 years ago. The finest dates come from Arabia and North Africa, for though American dates may be larger they lack the flavour of African and Asian varieties, where *compost* and not artificial fertilisers are used. Fresh dates contain vitamin B and counteract beri-beri. Arabs eat fresh dates but they also dry, grind and reduce them to flour from which they make a kind of bread, and throughout Arab countries 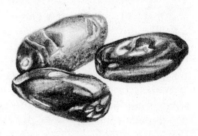 it is forbidden to cut down date trees without permission, for not only the fruit, but every part of the tree is used. The fruit is a fine source of energy and contains 20% water, 2.10% protein, 2.80% fat, 70.00% carbohydrates, and 1.60% mineral salts, mainly potassium.

Deafness. In the past there was no cure for deafness, which is usually caused by the thickening of the bones inside the ear. *D. D. Palmer*, however, cured deafness by means of *chiropractic*, *Ellis Barker* by *homeopathy* and recently many stubborn cases have been cured by *acupuncture, diet, fasting* and *vitamin* therapy.

Drs H. W. Bau and L. Savitt have cured patients of both tinnitus and nerve deafness by injecting them with 50,000 units of *vitamin A* daily, and in the Soviet Union fasts up to 14 days have restored the hearing of many who were thought to be incurable. There is also psychological deafness, which afflicts some who become convinced that they cannot hear. This can usually be cured by *hypnosis*.

Dermatitis. Derived from the Latin *derma*, skin and *itis*, inflammation. The word is loosely applied to a score of skin diseases, a few of which can be cured by the application of ointments. Those that resist orthodox means can usually be cured by *fasting*, a method used by *naturopaths* for the past 80 years or more. In 1970 Professor Ruben Babayants, an eminent physician in Moscow, gave details of his treatment, recorded in *Moskovsky Komsomolets*, in which he cured psoriasis, different kinds of eczema

41

and nettle rash by fasting patients from seven to 20 days, then putting them on diluted fruit juices, followed by undiluted juices, and finally on fruit, vegetables and dairy produce. No relapses were recorded. This merely confirms the experience of *naturopaths*, who are still scorned by the medical profession. *Vitamin* therapy, *homeopathy* and *acupuncture* have also been very successful in treating skin diseases.

Some skin diseases are caused by emotional stress, and these are often cured by *hypnotism* and psychiatry. See: Soap.

Decay, Dental. See: Caries.

De la Warr, George. Pioneer in Britain of radionics. He worked on the now established theory that there is a basic force in the universe, not limited by time or space, which radiates from everything, animate and inanimate. *Radionics* is a science which deals instrumentally with the radiations of all forms of matter but more especially with human radiations.

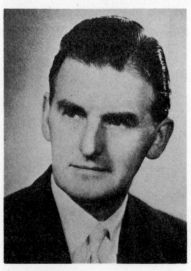

George de la Warr and his wife Marjorie, began their original research into energy fields in 1942 and during the course of this invented the radionic camera. They also invented other instruments embodying sonic vibration, magnetics and colour for physical treatment. They worked as a team till George de la Warr's death in 1969.

His theories, once scoffed at, are now gradually being accepted by scientists and medical men, and thousands of sufferers all over the world have benefited from radionic therapy. His work is now being carried on by his wife

George de la Warr

and colleagues at the De la Warr laboratories in Raleigh Park Road, Oxford. See: Radionics.

Detergents. Advertisements tell us that detergents contain *enzymes*; that they are the products of living organisms and hence are classified as biological material. But enzymes are not living creatures and according to Dr M. L. H. Flindt of the

Department of Occulational Health, Manchester University, enzyme dust causes severe bronchial ailments in factory workers*. The enzymes act as a sensitising agent and after repeated exposures to them workers developed *allergies*, some so violent that the victims thought they were going to die. Housewives can also suffer from asthma and skin diseases after using detergents, and because of this Mr Richard Sharples, Minister of State at the Home Office in 1971, ordered that the following warning should be printed on each packet: 'After each wash, rinse your hands and dry them thoroughly. People with sensitive or damaged skin should pay particular attention to the instructions for use and avoid prolonged contact with the washing solution.'

Rubber gloves should be worn, but the rubber now manufactured contains some chemical ingredient which brings out a rash on the hands of some who wear them.

Diabetes. There are two kinds of diabetes: *diabetes mellitus* (sweet) and *diabetes insipidus* (tasteless). Diabetes is derived from the Greek word *dia*, through, and *betes*, flowing, moving, because in both types the patient passes abnormal quantities of urine. *Mellitus* is the kind most common, the other being extremely rare.

It is a degenerative disease, mainly of the pancreas, which produces insulin, and when this is pumped into the blood it enables the body to utilise the sugar in food, and failure of the pancreas to do this causes diabetes. The malfunctioning of the liver is also thought to contribute to diabetes; and so do the emotions, which affect the secretion of hormones. Unless it has reached the final stages diabetes can be treated by *fasting*, *diet hydrotherapy*, *homeopathy* and herbal treatment. Many diabetics have been aided by *acupuncture*, and *osteopathy* and *chiropractic* also helps; but once the body has become entirely dependent on insulin, other methods have less chance of success.

Diet. Faulty diet is the main cause of most diseases, especially the degenerative ones. The food we eat is converted into blood, which nourishes all the organs. If the balance of blood is upset due to wrong feeding, one or more of the major organs or glands fail to function as they should, and disease starts.

Some insist on a vegetarian diet; others eat meat as well, but both kinds of diet, if properly balanced, are conducive to health.

*The Lancet: 14th June 1969

The main essential is to eat whole foods as pure as they can be bought. It is best, if possible, to grow your own fruit and vegetables in *compost* or humus, without the aid of sprays or artificial fertilisers; food that is not unduly processed and to which harmful chemicals and dyes have not been added, because health starts in the soil.

Food falls into five essential categories: *(a)* proteins *(b)* fats *(c)* carbohydrates *(d)* mineral salts *(e)* vitamins. One should consume them in roughly the right proportions: 15% protein, 5% fats, 20% carbohydrates, 60% fruit and vegetables. All types of food contain water. There is no need to worry about mineral salts or vitamins as they exist in fresh fruits, vegetables, nuts, dairy products, fish and in some kinds of meat. If any government had the courage to ban the sale of white flour and make *wholewheat* compulsory; ban white sugar, and advise people to eat less *salt,* the incidence of disease could be cut by half. These are 'dead' foods which, if eaten daily, tend to produce *diabetes, constipation,* headaches, rheumatism, etc., and after middle age, lassitude and dimness of sight and impaired hearing.

Digestion. Digestion is a complicated process, even now not fully understood. The body consists of about 60% water and the tissues, where chemical activity takes place, about 70% water. Most foods, however, are insoluble in water and must be broken down before they can pass through the walls of the small intestine and into the blood stream; so everything we eat has to be reduced before it can be utilised by the body cells, a process called *metabolism.*

Digestion starts in the mouth where teeth break food into pieces small enough to be swallowed and here it is mixed with dextrins and maltose by a ferment in the saliva called ptyalin. Unless well masticated the process will be incomplete and indigestion will result. Food passes from the mouth down the oesophagus to the stomach where it remains from one to five hours, depending on the kind of food eaten.

The stomach maintains food at a regular temperature; macerates, sterilises and digests the proteins and secretes a substance connected with the absorption of vitamin B12. It then passes into the small intestine where it is worked on by *enzymes, acids,* etc., to breakdown proteins and fats and digest them. Then it is absorbed into the small intestine, passes into the large intestine and finally into the bloodstream. The digestive system is a complicated and efficient factory for breaking down and processing food so that it can pass into the bloodstream; and the kinds of food we eat, and their combinations, either aid or inhibit this process.

Indigestible foods include new bread, buns, muffins, crumpets, hot and buttered; milk gulped down without being mixed with food; all fried foods; waxy potatoes; pastry and heavy fruit and suet puddings; unripe coarse fruit; nuts, lentils, sweets and chocolate; *strong* tea and coffee; alcoholic drinks; aerated waters.

Experiments carried out by two doctors working in 1931 revealed that it takes ¾ hour to digest a pint of water, 6½ hours a pint of milk, 2½ hours for two lightly boiled eggs, 1½ hours for two ounces of cane sugar, 4 hours for 4 oz boiled beef; 2½ hours for a vegetable salad, 4½ hours for 4 oz banana, 3¾ hours for 4 oz white bread, 6 hours for 4 oz butter, 4 hours for 5 oz potato. They found that the time of digestion depended not so much on the quantity of food eaten as on the amount of fat it contained*.

It is impossible to lay down hard and fast rules about food. For no apparent reason some foods suit one digestion and not another and it is a mistake, for instance, to force a child to eat food that is repugnant to him on the principle that 'it is good for you.' Fatty meat, sago pudding and lumpy porridge fall within this category. The *mind* and *taste* play an important part in digestion, and foods that look, smell and appear inviting make the digestive juices flow easily.

Diverticulitis. According to Mr Neil Painter, senior surgeon at Manor House Hospital, diverticular disease is the most common abnormality of the colon in the Western world, and 35% of British people over 60 are affected by it. In the past orthodox treatment was a bland diet, low in roughage; but it has now been proved that a bland diet is the *cause* of this disease, and fresh fruit and vegetables and wholewheat products to which are added miller's *bran,* a cure for it. Surgeon Captain T. L. Cleave was able while serving on the battleship George V during the Second World War, to cure stubborn constipation caused by a lack of fresh food, by giving *bran*. Mr Denis Burkitt, a surgeon with many years experience in Africa, found that rural Africans who eat bulky fibrous foods, rarely suffer from constipation, appendicitis and bowel cancer and that diverticulitis was rarely observed until the turn of the century when white flour came into wide use. *MacCarrison, Weston Price* and many other

* Reported in The Lancet – January 1931.

medical men found this out long before, and *Ellis Barker* and a host of food reformers were saying so even earlier, but few medical men would listen to them.

Dried Fruits. Very good 'energy foods', for they are concentrated. It takes about seven pounds of apricots, for instance, to produce one pound of dried fruit, and they are much better value than canned fruit. During dehydration fruit retains most of its vitamin B but loses much of its vitamin C, but the equivalent weights have far more calories and mineral salts. Dried fruits should be soaked in water from 16-20 hours, then heated to 100°F, but never boiled or excessively heated as they lose much of their natural flavour. Most dried fruits are rich in potassium, iron, phosphorus, sulphur, sodium and silicon.

Drown, Dr Ruth. A chiropractor in Los Angeles who improved and refined the Abrams Box and developed a camera to photograph the organs and tissues of patients, using nothing but a drop of blood, even though the subjects were miles away. It took pictures in cross section, which cannot be achieved by X-rays. Though this pioneer of *radionics* was granted a British patent for her apparatus her claim was denounced by the FDA in America as originating in the realms of science fiction and her equipment was confiscated. She was stigmatised in *Life Magazine* as a charlatan and died of grief, but left behind *Theory and Techniques of Radio Therapy*, probably the first book in the English language on the subject. Her work was carried on by G. W. Wigglesworth and his brother, in Chicago, who were electronics engineers. They developed an improved device known as a 'pathoclast' or disease-breaker and founded the Pathometric Association. See: Radionics.

Drugs. There is rarely need for the normal healthy person who falls ill to resort to drugs because a cure can be found by natural means. There are literally thousands of drugs on the market, most of which have side effects and many lead to addiction. Drugs aim at 'instant' results and often do considerable damage. Even so-called 'harmless' sleeping pills eventually fail to bring relief and as time goes on more have to be taken to obtain the same result. Herbal infusions, such as valerian, are more effective and have no side effects. Drugs are now Big Business into which thousands of millions of pounds have been sunk and no government has the courage or power to suppress the multinational companies who now control a good deal of medical thinking. They inundate doctors with advertisements and free samples and try to bring pressure on them to prescribe their products. In 1961 the Committee of Public Accounts informed Mr Enoch Powell, then Minister of Health, that manufacturers spent £6,500,000 to advertise their products, and a doctor in Tynemouth stated that in one week he received 235 packets of sample drugs weighing 14 lb, whjch cost £2.2/– in postage. The health of the country has deteriorated rather than improved by the spate of drugs. That is why those who hanker after health are weaning themselves off drugs and on to natural foods.

Duck's Egg. Duck's egg is easily infected by salmonella microbes and should never be eaten raw, or even lightly boiled. The only safe method is to cook the egg right through otherwise salmonella poisoning may result.

Dyed Foods. See: Chemicals in Food.

E

E Vitamin. See: Vitamin E.

Eddy, Mary Baker. (1821-1910). Born in Bow, Connecticut, Concord, USA, the sixth child of Congregational parents. Though illness limited her early education she read widely and wrote poetry. She suffered from a spinal disease, became preoccupied with questions of health and experimented with osteopathy. Then she heard of Phineas Quimby, who wrought remarkable cures without medicines or surgery, and was restored to health by him. This convinced her that Quimby had re-discovered the healing methods of Jesus, so she studied his notes and lectured on his theories. After Quimby's death she had a bad fall and medically was judged incurable. She turned to the New Testament, which she studied and regained health. That was the start of Christian Science. Students flocked to her and her fortunes improved. She published *Science and Health* which was enlarged to *Science and Health With a Key To The Scriptures*. In 1877 she married (for the third time) Asa A. Eddy, one of her disciples and founded the *Christian Science Journal, Christian Science Sentinal* and a daily paper, *Christian Science Monitor*.

Egg. The hen's egg is a food of high biological value, a good source of protein, and easily digested. The real value of eggs is that they can be made into so many palatable dishes, eaten in so many forms, and cooked so rapidly. The egg contains 73.70% water, 12.55% protein, 12.10% fat, 0.55% carbohydrates, and

1.10% mineral matter, being rich in phosphorus, sodium and potassium. It also contains vitamins A, B$_1$ and C. Custard powders contain no egg but consist mainly of starch dyed yellow, usually with turmeric, to give them a golden colour.

Elder *(Sambuccus nigra)*. The most undervalued of shrubs, which grows to a height of about four metres and is found all over Europe. Every part of the plant has medicinal uses and a tea made from the inner bark will get rid of the most stubborn *constipation*.

Elderberry. See: Berries, Elderberry.

Elderflower. The cream coloured flowers contain etheric oil, *rutin*, quercetin, glycosids, cholin, etc. Infused and mixed with honey they clear the skin and remove wrinkles and blemishes. Infused and taken as a tea they are a remedy for catarrh, coughs and colds, and bring relief if inflamed eyes are bathed in it. The infusion taken hot, with peppermint and yarrow, is a specific for colds and influenza, and will sometimes relieve asthma when all else has failed. An ointment made from the blossoms will relieve burns and banish scars. Elderflower wine is the prince of home-made wines and the superior of many costly white wines.

Emotions. Emotions affect the mind, cause the secretion of hormones into the blood and result in *psychosomatic* diseases. It has been shown that when under stress before an important event, an excess of sugar is discharged into the bloodstream, causing temporary *diabetes*. The right sort of emotions can maintain and improve health; the wrong sort can produce disease. Emotions are infectious. *Laughter*, for instance, produces laughter, and the gloom of one may affect others. This applies also to tears, anger, rage, etc.

Envy, jealousy, anxiety, deep sorrow, constant fear, and all evil emotions poison the bloodstream, whereas a happy state of mind, contentment and laughter bring health. In order to cultivate health it is necessary to think kind and pleasant thoughts, to try to forgive those who harm us, and cultivate a tolerant and sympathetic attitude. Over the years strong emotions etch themselves on the human face and bear witness to character.

Enzyme. Derived from the Greek *enzumos,* leavened; a substance of vegetable or animal origin, capable of producing chemical transformations, such as fermentation or oxidation; first found in yeast. Enzymes are also called ferments because those in yeast cause fermentation, frothing and bubbling due to the breakdown of carbohydrate into alcohol and carbon dioxide. Like all catalysts, they are not used up in the reaction. Enzymes produced in the body bring about chemical reactions rapidly and completely, whereas similar reactions outside the body are much more difficult to bring about and take far longer. How Nature's factory produces these miracles is not yet understood.

Exercise. Exercise is necessary for health. It helps to keep the joints and limbs supple, drives the blood to the furthermost ends of the body, and strengthens muscles and bones. It may be carried out in many ways: work, repetitive movements, athletics and games. All types of exercise are good. During work one exercises without conscious effort till weary. During repetitive movements the mind concentrates but the process is monotonous and comparatively few continue exercising for any length of time. The best form of exercise is games: indoor or outdoor, preferably the latter, in fresh air and sunshine. Games, provided they are not fiercely competitive, give pleasure, provide mental stimulus, are relaxing, and the finest of all forms of exercise. Because exercise increases respiration it dissipates fatigue by filling the lungs with oxygen; and the main cause of fatigue is lack of oxygen. The muscles are made up of protein, a substance comprising carbon, hydrogen, nitrogen and oxygen, together with traces of other elements. They contain a store of glycogen, a starch-like substance, which readily breaks down into sugar. Glycogen is the fuel which muscles need for their activity, and is used up during work. Another substance in muscle is lactic acid, which is liberated when muscles contract, causing fatigue. During a race of 100 metres about an ounce of lactic acid forms and the function of oxygen is to remove it. That is why one breathes much harder when fast and furious exercise is taken, or when very heavy work is done, such as lifting weights or moving heavy furniture. The oxygen inhaled recharges the generator.

Sugar, whether *dried fruit,* white or brown sugar, *honey* or *molasses,* taken shortly before a race, produces 'instant' energy, but in excess, sugar of any sort overloads the liver, produces fat, breaks down the kidneys and causes disease.

Eyes. The eyes are the most important organs of the body for without sight a man loses his independence. The eyes are not organs separate from the body, as so many imagine. They are nourished by *blood,* as are all the other organs. The eyes reflect the condition of the body and a science (iridology) has developed by which disease can be diagnosed by the condition of the eyes; for instance, the amputation of a limb will cause a spot to appear on a certain part of the iris. The first to discover this was a Hungarian Ignatz von Peczely, whose pet owl once buried its talons so deeply in one of his arms that its leg had to be amputated to release the talons. At the exact moment of the amputation he saw a tiny opening form in the iris of one of the bird's eyes. Later Peczely studied surgery and observed that whenever a limb was amputated a vacuole appeared in the patient's iris. He wrote a paper on the subject on which Dr Fortier-Bernoville founded the science of iridology.

A considerable amount of eye disease is caused either by faulty diet of the mother before birth, or is hereditary. The following diseases also affect the eyes: syphilis, small pox, diphtheria, measles, septicaemia, *rheumatism*, gonorrhoeal rheumatism, kidney disease, *diabetes,* tuberculosis, gout and malaria. Indigestion, *constipation* and headaches also cause eye trouble; and dental *caries* and weak eyes often run in harness. Eye teeth usually affect the eyes by the development of pyorrhoea at the roots. It has now been accepted that diabetes and cataract go hand in hand, and unless it has progressed too far, cataract often clears up if *diabetes* is cured. Heavy smoking may cause a form of blindness known as tobacco *amaurosis.*

Myopia, one of the commonest of eye afflictions, is usually associated with extremely poor health between birth and 16, especially severe illness during infancy.

Provided the light is good, reading small print will not harm the eyes. Sun glasses should be worn only when glare is unbearable, a rare condition in Britain. A sun vizor or eye shade is preferable, for the eyes were designed to accommodate sunshine. Constantly wearing dark glasses, especially at night or indoors, harms the eyes.

Many eye troubles are caused by *stress* and in the case of some myopics the belief that they cannot see objects at a distance, causes psychological short sight. Except when they are diseased most eye troubles can be cured by *exercise;* and some vanish when the diseases that cause them are cured. See: Bates.

F

Fasting. Most people confuse fasting with starving. Fasting is abstaining from food and is a health measure grafted into most of the ancient religions. Starvation comes from the Old English word *steorfan* which means 'to die a lingering death from hunger, cold, grief, or slow disease.' Almost everyone eats too much and when ill, people are urged to eat 'to keep up their strength'; but illness is often caused by overloading the digestive organs and fasting gives these a rest.

No animal can be forced to eat when ill. Only human beings stuff themselves. Food reformers have believed in the efficacy of fasting for nearly a century, and the yogis, Ancient Greek, Roman, Egyptian and Chinese physicians have recommended it. With characteristic thoroughness the Russians have done research into fasting and claim that skin diseases such as eczema, nettle rash and even psoriasis can be cured by fasts. They say that fasting helps to restore the balance of the hormones in the organism, and fasts of one day a month may extend the life span from two and a half to four and a half years. In Russian clinics patients are fasted for a multitude of diseases ranging from psychosis to bronchial asthma, stomach ulcers and diabetes. During fasts for up to 40 days the patient is given only diluted fruit juices or water. Fasts are broken by *fruit juices*, then fruit, vegetables and dairy produce. Men have fasted for more than 200 days without dying but fasts for more than two or three days should be undertaken only under the supervision of a naturopath – not an orthodox physician. Naturopaths have years of experience behind them, and with few exceptions doctors are new in this field.

There are exceptions and the list includes *Drs T. B. Allinson, Reginald Austin*, Sir V. Zachary Cope, the famous surgeon, Dr A. Eisdell More, Dr Allan Cott and many others; and in Russia Professor Pyotr Anokhin, Professor Ruben Babayants and Professor Vladimir Kikitin. Thousands of celebrities and ordinary citizens in Britain have benefited from fasting and diet reform at 'health farms' pioneered by men like *Stanley Lief* and *James Thomson*, including Churchill, E. M. Trelawny Irving, Yehudi Menuhin and *Mahatma Gandhi*, who was a consistent faster. In America fasting was given a great boost by *Bernarr Macfadden* and the *Kelloggs*. In his autobiography *Yesterday*, the writer Robert Hichens, says that for many years he had a 'tea day' each week, during which he ate nothing. Hichens lived to top 90. I also used to fast one day each week but, with the advance of age I eat far less and fast only once a fortnight or three weeks – and always if I feel out of sorts. After a short fast one feels more mentally and physically alert, a feeling only those know who have fasted.

Fats. Fats are substances that cannot be dissolved in water but are soluble in liquids such as paraffin, chloroform, ether, etc., which are known as fat-solvents. Fats differ widely: some such as butter and lard are solid under normal conditions but liquefy when heated. When fat is eaten it is broken down by fatty acids and glycerol in the digestive system, partly by saponification and partly by *enzymes*. Because of this only fats and oils capable of saponification should be used as food. Mineral oils, such as liquid paraffin, cannot be saponified and when consumed deprive the body of its store of *vitamin A*, and tend to cause cancer.

Some fats, such as *butter*, contain vitamins A, D, and a little C. So do most vegetable oils, unless they have been hydrogenated and processed, when the *vitamin C* is destroyed.

Weight for weight fats provide twice as much energy as *carbohydrates* and on reaching the tissues are burnt as fuel and help to keep us warm. Without fats the nervous system would deteriorate. Unfortunately, if more fat is eaten than is needed it is stored in the liver and under the skin; in women more easily than men. That is why they resist the cold better than men.

Women, who in their determination to slim eat only *protein* and eschew fat, defeat themselves, for by a complicated process the ferments in the liver destroy the amino-acids and the residue is changed either into glucose or fatty acid; so some carbohydrate should be taken with protein at the same meal. Fortunately all vegetable protein foods contain a substantial proportion of carbohydrates.

Feet. The feet get more heavy use than any part of the body for whether running, walking or standing the weight is borne by them. Though 90% of people are born with perfect feet 8% develop foot trouble in the first year and 41% in the first five years. By the age of twenty 80% suffer from minor foot troubles and few reach 50 without experiencing them. Foot troubles are usually caused by badly designed or 'fashionable' footwear. The most common causes are: (1) bad posture (2) wrong way of walking (3) ill-fitting footwear (4) standing for too long, or in the wrong posture, or on concrete or marble floors (5) faulty *diet*. Bad posture throws the spinal column out of line, irritates the spinal nerves which radiate to all parts of the body and causes a multitude of ailments from headaches and stomach ulcers to *rheumatism*. Feet should be washed night and morning, nails should be pared and cleaned, and socks should be changed daily. Bad feet lead to bad health. The designers of platform soles and stiletto heels should be put out of business.

Fig. Since ancient times the fresh fig has been regarded as one of the finest foods for the convalescent. Figs increase strength in the young, preserve the elderly and make them look younger and less wrinkled. In ancient Greece and Rome figs were a staple food and they were held in high esteem by the Egyptians, Hebrews and Hindus. They are a good source of *riboflavin* and thiamin, *vitamins C* and *A*, are rich in *iron*, *copper* and *calcium* and contain a protein-digesting enzyme called ficin or cradein. When figs are dried the vitamin content is negligible but the amount of natural sugar increases by about 65% and they are among the finest natural laxatives. Fresh figs contain 79% water, 1.50% protein, 0.20% fat, 18.70% carbohydrates and 0.60% mineral matter. Smyrna dried figs contain 18.80% Water, 4.30% protein, 0.30% fat, 74.20% carbohydrates and 2.40% mineral matter.

Finsen, Neils (1860-1904). Danish scientist who, by observing the movements of a cat on a roof, which constantly moved into the sun as the shadows crept over it, realised that in sunlight there is some element which benefits living creatures. By constantly experimenting he used plain sunlight, and then sunlight through coloured glass, to kill tuberculosis bacilli and cure *skin* complaints. His work was taken up and advanced by others, notably *Rollier*, Strandberg and Gauvin. See: Sun bathing.

Fish. Fish is an excellent source of protein and can be divided into 'fat' and 'lean' fish. Fat fish, such as bloaters, herrings, kippers, sardines, sprats and whitebait contain about 10% or more of fat;

eels 15% and salmon about 13.0% Fish is one of the best sources of *nicotinic acid,* and fat fish a good source of *vitamins A* and *D.* The protein in fish ranges from 18.00% in cod to 22.00% in haddock and halibut. As fish does not contain carbohydrates, lean fish is ideal for slimmers. It is also a good and easily digested food for the very young, the very old and dyspeptics. Despite what many people imagine, fish play no part in a vegetarian diet.

Fletcherism. Horace Fletcher, an American, propounded the theory that ill health is caused by faulty digestion due to unmasticated food. He chewed each mouthful 33 times till the food was liquified in his mouth, before swallowing it, enabling ptyalin and other gastric juices to break it down and prepare it for the *enzymes* in the *stomach* and intestines. He restored his own broken health and for a few years had a considerable following. Thousands paid tribute to Fletcherism as the cure for all ailments. Though thorough mastication is necessary, Fletcherism is now considered a cranky theory.

Flower Wines. Though alcoholic, flower wines have medicinal properties. If properly made they do not contain chemicals and leave no hangover, are easy to make and cheap when compared with commercial vintages. The *alcohol* created by fermention, is necessary to preserve the flower essences. Cowslip wine will cure jaundice, *dandelion* is good for the *digestion* and *kidney* trouble, sloe wine effectively stops diarrhoea. *Elderberry* wards off colds and coughs and makes a fine warming winter drink, *blackcurrant* is good for *colds* and *bronchitis, barley* is good for the *kidneys,* and *apple* a fine all-round health drink. Rhubarb, though a palatable wine, is bad for *rheumatism.*

Fluorite. One of the many minerals found in the body and a principal acid-forming element. The body of a 150 lb man contains two ounces. In nature it exists chiefly in fluospar and calcium fluoride. Traces of fluorite occur in many minerals, in some water, the bones of mammals, and in the enamel of teeth. Traces are found in nearly all plants and animals; in the blood of birds and mammals; in the yolks of eggs and in milk, where it is combined with fat; and in the outer coats of grains. It is necessary for the formation of the enamel on the teeth and the development of the skeleton. No bony substance can be formed without it. A deficiency of fluorite in the lens of the eye is followed by ophthalmic disease.

Folic Acid. About 35 years ago researchers into the complex B vitamins fed a deficient diet to monkeys which was similar to the nutritionally low diet of the very poor in India and they developed an anaemic condition as well as a bone disease. The disease was relieved by giving them an extract of yeast, confirming the fact that there is an active substance in yeast which cures some types of anaemia. Day issued a report on the subject and later Williams, Mitchell and Snell discovered that this substance existed also in green leaves and vegetables, liver, kidney, *mushrooms* and wheat bran. They called it folic acid and Koch and Spies used folic acid for the treatment of macrocytic anaemia in humans. Shortly after treatment they noticed a significant increase in the haemoglobin and red blood cells and the patients felt stronger and put on weight. It is now known that folic acid is necessary for the maintenance of the normal number of red blood cells, for aid in liver activity and for many functions of the endocrine glands. It is essential for protein *digestion,* for the utilisation of *calcium* and *iron* and pantothenic acid. See: Vitamin B.

Food Reform. Often confused with vegetarianism, but many reformers include milk products in their diet, and some flesh and fish. Food should be balanced; that is, essential foods should· be eaten in roughly the right proportions.

Diet is an art and not a complete science. Allowances must be made for individual preferences. Hippocrates said: 'An inferior diet liked by the patient is preferable to a superior diet which he dislikes.' Our taste buds make us like one food and dislike another. Some cannot abide milk, others fat; acid fruits disagree with many and sago pudding is anathema to most children. It is no use telling them to 'Eat up; it will do you good,' for one person's meat may be another's poison. Thomas Cogan (1545-1607), a wise physician, wrote: 'Custom bringeth liking, and liking causeth good concoction. For what the stomach liketh, it greedily desireth; and having received it, closely encloseth it about until it is duly concocteth. Which thing is the cause that meat and drink wherein we have great delight, though it be much worse than the other, yet it does us more good.'

That is why so many flourish on foods that are designated as harmful by dieticians and doctors. See: Smell, Taste.

Frozen Foods. For more than 4,000 years it has been known that edibles deteriorate and putrefy in the warm but keep fresh for considerable periods in the cold. King Solomon sent slaves into the mountains for ice which he packed round fruit and other comestibles, and vessels in which wine was stored. When the Arctic Circle was explored hunters found the frozen carcases of mammals lying in packed ice, which were edible. From the start of the 20th century cold storage has been used to an increasing degree, till today all imported meat is frozen and turkeys that do not sell at Christmas are kept till the following season – sometimes for two or three years. Frozen mutton retains its structure practically unchanged when thawed, but beef loses a large amount of muscle cell fluids or meat juice when thawed; both can be kept for many months without apparent deterioration. Fish is frozen at much lower temperatures than meat and if stored at 10°F below freezing may remain untainted for as long as eight months. Eggs in cold storage soon develop a musty flavour and produce *bacteria,* which ruins them as food. Fruit and vegetables are usually stored in inert gases, which inhibit the ripening process.

Francis Bacon was the first Englishman to preserve food scientifically, which he did one bitter March day in 1626, when he emerged from his coach in Highgate, bought a fowl and stuffed it with snow. Unfortunately, he caught a cold in the process and died within a fortnight.

Three hundred years later Clarence Birdseye, who was studying game and fish in Northern Labrador for the US Biological Survey, found that when thawed, frozen fish and venison were as tasty as when fresh. He reproduced the process in his Massachusetts laboratory and founded the quick-frozen foods industry. Today food is frosted at fast temperatures well below zero F., the temperature varying according to the product, and then transported in refrigerators to the point of sale and displayed in shops at zero temperature. Placed in household refrigerators at 40–50°F frozen food will keep for a week or ten days, and it is claimed that when defrosted these foods taste better than 'fresh' foods displayed in the shops, which may have been picked many days earlier. Such a claim does not bear examination for the finest flavours come from foods picked and eaten on the same day.

Quick-freezing destroys *vitamin C* in fruit and vegetables and there are dangers connected with the eating of meat and fish once they have been defrosted and returned to the refrigerator. They may then breed bacteria rapidly and have caused thousands of cases of food poisoning.

The idea that milk placed in the cold chamber of a refrigerator will keep indefinitely, is a mistaken one. The US Department of Agriculture (1933) stated that high quality raw milk started with 31,000 microbes per c.c., contained four times that number after 24 hours, and the same milk, if left for 1½ hours at 75°F generated 10½ times that number of microbes. Convenience foods, which depend upon refrigeration, are a permanent feature of modern life. They are safe provided suitable precautions are taken. See: Germs, Bacteria, Microbes.

Fruitarian. Term applied to one who lives almost exclusively on fruit and nuts. There are thousands of fruitarians in India, a colony in Germany, and a number in America and Britain. As long ago as 1901 Professor Jaffa of the US Department of Agriculture, issued a dietary study of a family which had lived on a diet limited to fruit and nuts for seven years without harming their health in any way. They added celery, honey, olive oil and occasionally a small amount of prepared cereals to their diet, and ate only two meals a day: one at 10.30 and the other at 5.00 in the afternoon. On an average day they consumed 33 grammes of protein food and 150 grammes of carbohydrates, the total fuel value amounting to 1,300 calories. They weighed less than normal for people of their stature but, according to Jaffa they were all – even a girl of 13 – extremely active. She ate 26 grammes of protein, 52 of fat and 157 of carbohydrates, with a calorific value of 1,235 a day, and seemed extremely fit. He commented: 'Not withstanding the facts brought out by this comparison, the subject had the appearance of a well-fed child in excellent health and spirits.' In the same year the accepted dietary standard for a child of 13, and of average activity, called for 90 grammes of *protein* and amounted to 2,450 calories.

While it is possible to live on a fruitarian diet it is inadvisable to do so, for taste and variety are important factors in diet and one should take advantage of the prodigality of Nature. Green leafy foods are rich in vitamins and minerals; beans and legumes are rich in proteins, and milk products add richness and variety. In Britain a fruitarian diet would be too costly for most people. See Diet.

Fruit Juices. With the invention of electrical juice extractors it is now possible to supplement one's diet with fruit and vegetable juices, which are rich in minerals and vitamins and water of the purest kind, which is filtered through the trunks and stems of trees and plants.

Man was never meant to live on concentrated fruit juices, however, and fruit juice should always be diluted with water. Large quantities of concentrated juices will eventually overload the kidneys. Fruit and vegetable juices are valuable when taken diluted during fasts. See: Fasting.

G

G-Vitamin. See: Vitamin G.

Gandhi, M. K. (Mahatma). Mahatma Gandhi, the Father of Modern India, was an inveterate experimenter who tried to discover the cheapest and most nutritious *diet* on which the poor in India could live in perfect health. Though born into a family of vegetarians he tried early in life to eat goat's flesh to see what it was like, and was nauseated. When he came to Britain to study for the Bar he was told by British friends that it was impossible to maintain health in a cold climate on fruit and vegetables and that meat was essential to health. But he persisted and for some weeks lived on porridge, milk and wholewheat bread. Then he discovered a vegetarian restaurant in the City and eventually formed a vegetarian group and became a leading vegetarian.

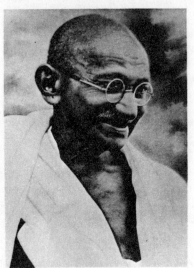
Mahatma Gandhi

Some years after his return to India he asked *Dr W. R. Aykroyd*, head of the Institute of Nutrition, Coonoor, South India, to collaborate with him in experiments on food. He was interested chiefly in obtaining protein foods from leaves and grass, cheap enough for the poorest villager, and eventually between them they devised many suitable diets. Up to the time of his assassination he was deeply concerned with providing cheap, nourishing food for his countrymen and others learnt from his experiments, and the work he started is still progressing. He also wrote a practical little book called *Diet Reform* in which are given details of his experiments and his collaboration with *Dr Aykroyd*.

Garlic. Garlic has gained the reputation of being the Queen of the Cooking Herbs. The French consider, rightly, that cooking without garlic is inconceivable. The Italians, Spaniards and Slavs esteem it highly, and most Indian curries contain garlic. It is more than a fine cooking herb, however: it has medicinal properties and is an excellent health food. The Egyptians used it as long ago as 5,500 BC; Sanskrit literature praised its virtues 3,000 years ago; Pliny thought highly of it and made it the subject of a treatise he wrote in Salerno; and Nicholas Culpepper, the famous herbalist, recommended it as a specific for many ailments. The Israelite slaves ate 'garlick' when they were building the pyramids, and later in the wilderness (Numbers 11.5).

Garlic lends flavour to cooked food as no other ingredient does. It is rich in vitamins B, C and D and the minerals copper, zinc, aluminium, manganese, sulphur and iron and is one of the finest internal antiseptics known. In 1937 chemists at the University of Southern California analysed garlic and found it contained crotonic aldehyde, and during the Second World War Soviet doctors called it 'the Russian penicillin', as its action was similar to that of penicillin, with the advantage that garlic has no side effects, and no one is allergic to it.

During the Great Plague that swept Europe in the Middle Ages those who ate garlic seemed immune and the herb was 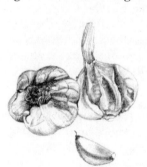 used to prevent the disease from spreading. Many modern physicians have experimented with garlic and found it to be an admirable specific. Dr W. C. Minchin who was in charge of a large tubercular ward in the Kells Hospital, Dublin, where incurables were sent, aroused interest by his claims to have cured TB by administering garlic in the form of inhalants, ointments and compresses. A contemporary, Dr M. W. McDuffie, also used garlic on 'incurable' patients in the Metropolitan Hospital, New York and achieved a number of remarkable cures. Americans and Russians who have done research on garlic find that it destroys harmful bacteria in the intestinal tract and increases beneficial bacteria; and Dr Piotrowski at the Geneva Hospital, stated in *Praxis* that garlic helps to reduce high blood pressure by dilating the blood vessels. In India it has been found that if cooked with other edibles garlic will preserve them for days at temperatures over 100°F.

Germs See: Bacteria.

Glands, Endocrine. Derived from the Greek *hormaein,* meaning to excite, urge, stimulate, which is what they do. They manufacture hormones which are secreted into the bloodstream. There are nine endocrine glands: pineal, pituitary, thyroid, parathyroid, thymus, the Islets of Langerhans, adrenals, ovaries, and testes. Their products or the lack of them, affect growth, the emotions and a great many other things. Some act very rapidly – almost instantly – whereas others take much longer. Though the effects of some glands were known more than 150 years ago, there is still much to be learnt about them.

Glucose. Glucose occurs naturally in fruits, some vegetables, *honey* and golden syrup, but there is also commercial glucose, which is a mixture of dextrins and glucose made by boiling starch with a strong acid, and is used largely in the manufacture of confectionery, squashes and 'fruit' drinks. Most people are under the impression that because commercial glucose is very easily digested it is good for one, and athletes often imbibe glucose drinks to give them 'instant energy'; but Dr Christopher Woodard, Honorary Consultant to British Olympic teams in 1948 and 1952 said: 'The best forms of sugar in order of digestibility are *brown sugar, honey,* treacle and *white sugar.* I do not recommend glucose because it usually gives fit men and women indigestion. It is, so to speak, a predigested form of sugar, and whereas it is all right for old ladies who cannot digest sugar for themselves, it is not the sort of thing that a normally fit person should need to take.'

Glucose is also condemned in an article by Margaret Lamb, LDS, in *The British Dental Journal:* 'For the body to use carbohydrates successfully *vitamin B* must be present and, if not supplied with the food as it is in natural sugar, then the vitamin is absorbed from the body's storage depots.

'Quite often on the labels of sweet jars, certain jams and jellies and invalid drinks, you read that the product is made with glucose – as though that were a virtue. Glucose is a synthetic product made by treating corn starch with hydrochloric or sulphuric acid, neutralising the resultant syrup with calcium carbonate and decolourising with carbon or bone black. According to Leo, the American nutritionist, glucose is the only known sugar to cause diabetes in animals.' This is endorsed in a Report by the Foods Standards Committee submitted to the Minister of Health in 1959.

Graham, Sylvester. One of the earliest advocates of wholewheat flour and bread in America, which was called 'Graham crackers'. He also wrote one of the earliest books on the subject: *Treatise on Bread.*

Grape. See: Berries, grape.

Grass. 'All flesh is grass,' said the Prophet Isaiah, 'and all the goodliness thereof is as the flower of the field,' not realising perhaps, how true, scientifically, were his words. Later Nebuchadnezzar, king of the Babylonians, withdrew from the haunts of men and 'ate grass like oxen.' There are more than 4,500 varieties of grass, many of them edible. Until recently it was considered food fit only for cattle and not till just after the First World War did the importance of grass as food for humans become apparent. In 1918 when the Austrian Army occupied Auronzo in Italy, they commandeered nearly all the food and the natives were forced to live for a year mainly on grass and hay – and there was not a single death in the village! When the Austrians were defeated and the people returned to their normal diet the death rate rocketed. Since then considerable research has been done on grass and in 1940 the chemists George O. Kohler, W. R. Graham and C. F. Schnabel, of Kansas City, Mo., discovered that grass contains all the vitamins known at the time except D, and is 28 times as rich in vitamins as most vegetables. They experimented with the leaves of wheat, barley, oats and rye and produced a fine white powder with a slightly malt flavour. They ate this powder all winter and enjoyed remarkable health, being singularly free from colds.

Dr Barbara Moore, a vegetarian, lived entirely on fruit, vegetable juices, nuts and grass clippings from Kensington Gardens and when well over the age of 50 performed feats of considerable endurance, on one occasion walking from Oxford to her home in London.

During the 1939-45 war J. R. Beadon Branson, a *food reformer* who lived on grass, fruit and raw vegetables, offered to teach commandos how to live on grass so that they could be independent of all other food. And a Ceylonese named Carolis, became famous because he lived for years exclusively on grass and plain water which he claimed gave him strength and unusual endurance.

Since then it has been proved that not only is grass rich in vitamins but that it contains protein of excellent quality, equal to that of meat and cheese. Its only drawback is that grass in large quantities is indigestible and a grass diet monotonous and tasteless. Small quantities of young grass chopped and eaten in salads, provide an excellent food supplement. Today milk, cream and cheese are made from grass, as well as milk chocolate, which looks and tastes like the genuine article, is much more easily digested and better for health.

H

Hahnemann, Samuel Christian (1755-1843). Founder of *homeopathy*, born in Meissen, Saxony. He obtained a medical degree in Vienna, became assistant to Dr Quarin, physician to the Empress Marie Theresa and during visits to prisons and ships realised how important a part environment played in health. His life changed when a *Materia Medica* by Cullen, an Englishman, fell into his hands. Pages were devoted to the new Peruvian bark *(cinchona)*, used to cure the Countess of Cinchon of a fever in Peru. He obtained some of the bark, took four drachms daily, and contracted the fever. When discontinued, the fever vanished. This made him think and he set about treating likes with likes *(similia similibus)* and later wrote an *Essay On The New Principle*, which maintained that disease could be cured only by substances which when taken in substantial doses

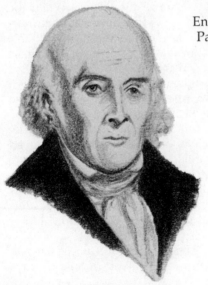

Sketch of Samuel Hahnemann taken from a portrait by Scheffer

would, in healthy persons, produce symptoms characteristic of the diseases they were supposed to heal. His theory was ridiculed and invective poured on his head. Then in 1799 he attended a family where three members were struck down by scarlet fever but a delicate daughter who succumbed to every illness, escaped. He learnt that she had been treated with belladonna for another disorder, so he prescribed tiny doses of belladonna for her sisters and brothers and cured them.

At first he used to administer only one substance at a time and called his system *homeopathy*, coined from the Greek *hominos*, like; and *pathos*, disease. In 1838 the government of Saxony ordered belladonna to be given to patients suffering from scarlet fever.

In 1810 he wrote *The Organon of the Rational Art of Healing* which was printed simultaneously in America. It was attacked by orthodox medical men but attracted scores of thinking physicians who flocked to Vienna to learn about the new art, and a school of homeopathy came into being.

His great triumph occurred in 1831 when a cholera epidemic broke out in Eastern Europe and thousands perished. He studied the symptoms and decided that camphor would cure the disease; his advice was accepted by the Cholera Commission and the epidemic was mastered. Hahnemann's fame spread and Dr F. F. Quin, Napoleon's Irish physician, became a convert and on his return to England founded the London Homeopathic Hospital. When in 1840 cholera swept Britain and 54,000 perished, it was found that 59.20% of those who died had been treated by orthodox methods whereas only 16.40% by homeopathy succumbed. Lord Ebury produced these figures when the Health Act came before the House of Lords and homeopaths were placed on the Register, for this and other evidence convinced the government of the value of the new treatment. See: *Homeopathy*.

Hay, Dr W. H. An orthodox medical man and a graduate of New York University, who shocked the medical profession when he advocated natural methods of healing and claimed that his famous 'Hay Diet' in which predominantly protein and carbohydrate food were not included in the same meals, cured illness and reduced weight. He was villified but his methods were so successful and he made so much money by books, lectures and articles that he could afford to defy the AMA. He was a firm believer in fasting as a means of curing disease, and the bane of specialists, who treat individual organs or parts of the body, instead of the body as a whole. He had disciples in every continent and many physicians agreed with him. Dr Morris of Detroit, for instance, said that when he sent patients to a group clinic he expected them to return with a diagnosis of every disease that was represented by the clinic as a whole. If a patient returned without a diagnosis of heart disease, he knew that the heart specialist must have been absent.

He was condemned for saying that carbohydrate and protein foods should be separated but there seems to be a modicum of truth in his theory for in 1924 when he was a member of a gymnasium class in Buffalo he organised an endurance test with a class of 18 men ranging in age from 28 to 55. For lunch they ate a predominantly starch meal and for dinner a predominantly protein meal and they were asked not to take their usual physical exercise during a four-week period. At the end of the first week their endurance showed, on average, a 50% increase and at the end of a month an increase of 165%. Hay maintained that endurance is decreased by an accumulation of acid end-products resulting from an incompatible mixture of protein and carbohydrate foods.

Hearing. Man is endowed by a sense of hearing to enable him to communicate easily. Hearing also enables one to avoid danger, and without hearing music could not be enjoyed, or dancing to its rhythms. With advancing age the bones and membranes of the inner ear thicken, nerves are affected and deafness supervenes, a process which can be arrested by eating the right foods in roughly the right proportions. A stodgy *diet* usually causes tinnitus due to the decay of the auditory nerve, and can be cured by B-complex vitamins, and C and A. Drs H. W. Bau and L. Savitt have cured cases of advanced deafness by giving patients 50,000 units of vitamin A daily, or 25,000 units of A together with brewer's yeast and pituitary extract three times a day. This, together with B-complex and C have proved remarkably effective. Naturopaths have also achieved remarkable results in some cases of *deafness* by fasting and *food reform*, and hypnotists have often cured 'psychological deafness'. See: Deafness.

Herbalism. The most ancient of all forms of healing. The British Museum has records of a herbal that belonged to the King of Assyria (668—626 BC) and Egyptian papyri circa 2,000 BC contain herbal recipes. The Ancient Hindus, Chinese, Persians, Aztecs, Greeks and Red Indians used herbal recipes; the Chinese 7,000 years ago and the Hindus even before that. Much of Hindu lore was handed down by word of mouth and one of the herbs they used – *rawolfia* – has only recently been rediscovered by scientists.

The public is now so cynical about the orthodox medical profession that herbalism has regained its former popularity for herbalists are curing many whom physicians fail to cure. The US Government, for instance, is paying for the training of medicine men at a special school in Rough Rock, Arizona and in 1972 the first six students graduated. Doctors in Britain are also investigating African methods and the ancient Hindu system of Ayurvedic medicine based on herbs, both of which have achieved cures after orthodox methods have failed. In China herbal medicine is used in conjunction with allopathy.

Originally all substances given to the sick were called drugs but today there is a difference between herbal medicines and drugs. In modern medicine drugs such as asprin and digitalis are manufactured from the active principle of *salix* (willow) and *digitalis* (foxglove), whereas herbalists use the entire herb, parts of which contain other healing elements. Drugs often have side-effects, herbs do not.

Hindhede, Professor Mikkel (1862-1945). A country doctor in Denmark who even as a young man had doubts about the suitability of foods normally consumed. He tried out all kinds of food on himself and then on his wife and four children over a number of decades, and questioned as unnatural such things as baldness, dental decay, goitre, cold feet and menstrual disorders in women which were accepted as normal. He established a minimum amount of protein necessary for health, which was less than half the amount advocated by doctors of his time.

When America entered the war in 1917 the Danes were placed in a serious position, for the foundation of their economy was based mainly on 5,000,000 domestic animals. Denmark, till then, had imported grain from America for humans and for animals. Professor Hindhede, Superintendent of the State Institute of Food Research, was appointed Food Adviser to the government. He decided to get rid of 75% of the pigs and let the people eat the grain that had fed them, not as bran mash but as wholewheat bread with coarse bran added. Distillation of spirits from grain and potatoes was stopped and only half the normal quantity of beer was brewed. The population lived mainly on vegetables, potatoes and grain.

As a result the death rate which had been 12.5 per thousand in 1913 fell to 10.4, the lowest registered in any European country.

The Danish diet consisted of wholewheat bread with added bran, green vegetables, potatoes, other root vegetables, fruit, milk and butter. Only the rich could afford meat (much less than before), which was scarce in towns, and little alcohol was consumed. The fall in the death rate and the vast improvement in the health of the nation – all within twelve months – was one of the most remarkable dietetic stories in the history of nations, and the world learnt that meat need not be a staple food. The lesson was forgotten soon after the war ended.

After the war a scurrilous campaign was launched by commercial interests to discredit his ideas but he defended his reputation in court and was granted a government pension of Kr. 6,000 a year on his 70th birthday for his services to the nation.

Homeopathy. A system of treatment based on the principle that 'like cures like', founded by *Hahnemann*. It is also a treatment traditionally observed by drinkers who, after heavy alcoholic sessions have been sobered the following morning by taking a little of the refreshment they indulged in the night before; that is 'a hair of the dog that bit them'.

Homeopathy does not treat patients in the conventional way by suppressing disease. It stimulates the body's own mechanism; and the patient is treated, not the disease.

There are more than 2,000 homeopathic medicines in use, derived from natural sources; some innocuous, others poisonous, including deadly nightshade and snake venom. The potency of homeopathic medicines is increased by *decreasing* the amount of substance in them. This, though seemingly paradoxical, seems to work. Drugs are prepared in two scales: decimal (divided by ten) and centesimal (divided by 100). Originally all solid matter was prepared by grinding it thoroughly in a mortar, a method known as trituration, which sometimes took an hour or more. Today machines do the work in seconds.

If, for instance, a homeopath prescribes sulphur, he puts a grain of sulphur into a mortar and adds nine grains of sugar of milk and triturates the mixture, which is considered to have a potency of Ix, x being the Latin for ten. I x is the first decimal potency.

If a higher potency is needed, nine grains of the new mixture are set aside and the remaining tenth grain mixed with nine grains of sugar of milk, and this is triturated to obtain the second decimal potency. By repeating the process, potencies of 3x, 4x, 5x, etc., are produced, each containing less and less of the original drug.

When trituration is employed the drug potentised becomes colloidal and is soluble in water and spirit. Very high potencies such as 200th, 1,000th and 10,000th which contain microscopic quantities of the drug are prepared by dilution in water or spirit or made into pills by moistening sugar pills with the dilution. In liquid form these are known as 'mother tinctures', and by the same process very high potencies can be produced. Accurate machines are made to measure and manufacture homeopathic remedies.

No homeopath will ever inject a live virus into the bloodstream and immunity against small-pox, for instance, is developed by placing a drug on the tongue (*variolimum*) which is so effective that when administered it is almost impossible to get a vaccination to take. Homeopathic remedies have no side-effects and no harmful after-effects.

Years ago the BMA appointed four eminent physicians to investigate and expose homeopathy. In due course three of them became homeopaths and the fourth failed to submit his report.

Homeopaths insist on their patients following food reform and many, such as the late *Ellis Barker,* that during treatment they follow a meatless diet. See: Hahnemann. Information may be obtained from, in Britain, the British Homeopathic Association Inc., 27a Devonshire St., London W.1. Telephone (01) 935 2163. In America, The National Center for Homeopathy, 6231 Loesburg Pike, Suite 506, Falls Church, Virginia 22044. Telephone (703) 534-4363.

Honey. A sweet viscid fluid, the nectar of flowers, collected and worked up for food by certain insects; bees throughout the world; ants in Australia. It contains about equal parts of glucose and fructose and is flavoured by small amounts of volatile substances derived from flowers. Honey from different areas may differ widely in flavour and aroma, depending on the flowers from which it is extracted, but the mean composition of honey is: moisture 17.70%, invert sugar 74.98%, sucrose 1.90%, dextrin 1.51%, ash 0.18%. English honey contains 0.40% protein, a trace of fat, 76.40% carbohydrates, no starch, and each pound produces about 1,320 calories. The sugar in honey exists in a predigested form and is ready for immediate assimilation and as such is a valuable form of instant energy.

Honey also contains 0.05 mg of riboflavin and 0.20 mg of nicotinic acid per 100 gm., and plant acids such as formic, citric, etc., various gums, oil and pollen, depending on the region in which the flowers grow. There are also traces of sodium, potassium, calcium, magnesium, iron, copper, phosphorus, sulphur and chlorine. Honey is superior in every respect to other forms of sweetening for it appears to contain some health-giving substance which has defied analysis.

It is a heart stimulant, is good for anaemia and haemorrhage, as it helps the blood to clot, builds resistance to coughs and colds, soothes burns, induces sleep, and is powerful enough to kill all micro-organisms introduced into it. It also has the power to absorb moisture from anything it comes into contact with, and as a result kills many virulent germs. Because of this it is used as a dressing in many British hospitals.

Honeycomb. The comb in which honey is manufactured by bees is an extremely accurately built structure for every angle in the hexagonal apertures is exactly 135 degrees. The comb consists of waxy substances which are probably incapable of being digested, though both honey and the comb can be eaten. There is some substance in the comb, which when thoroughly chewed and liberated, cures hay fever and asthma in many people. *Dr D. C. Jarvis* first propounded this theory in America and was scoffed at for being 'unscientific', but the writer was cured of hay fever which he suffered every June for 25 years, by chewing honeycomb, and has recommended the cure to others, with gratifying results, though why the chewing of the comb brings relief, not even Dr Jarvis knows.

Hopkins, Sir Frederick Gowland. He left school at 17 to become an insurance clerk but six months later started an apprenticeship as a chemical analyst and qualified with distinction. Was employed as an assistant at the Home Office till 1888 when a small legacy enabled him to enter Guy's Hospital Medical School. In 1898 he went to Cambridge to run the medical science course and in 1901 when the Dutch scientist Gerrit Grijns suggested that beri-beri might be caused by the absence of some factor missing in the diet eaten by the poor in the Dutch East Indies, which was mainly of polished rice, Hopkins experimented and found that rats fed on a diet of pure *protein, carbohydrates, fat* and *salt* failed to grow and lost weight unless given small quantities of milk, thus proving that accessory food factors or *vitamins,* as they were called later, were necessary for health. For this discovery he was knighted in 1925, awarded the Nobel Prize for medicine in 1929, and elected President of the Royal Society in 1931. He was instrumental in founding the science of medical biochemistry and at the time of his death no fewer than 75 of his former pupils held chairs in the subject all over the world.

Hormone. Chemical substance secreted by an endocrine gland and carried by the blood to another organ in which it initiates activity; generally used widely to include substances producing an inhibitory effect.

Howard, Sir Albert, CIE, MA. Famous for his research in agriculture. Went to India as Economic Botanist at the Agricultural Institute in Pusa, Bengal, where he learnt to grow healthy crops free from disease without the aid of artificial fertilisers, sprays, insecticides, fungicides and germicides. He proved at Pusa, and later at the Experimental Farm in Quetta, that animals fed on produce raised in *humus* do not contract foot-and-mouth disease, even when in close contact with sick animals. The lessons he learnt were published in numerous papers and books, among them *Farming and Disease*, but generally speaking his words have fallen on fallow ground for the manufacturers of fertilisers have too much at stake, and the government gains enormously from the taxes they pay, to heed Howard's theories. Animals are still slaughtered at the slightest hint of foot-and-mouth disease, instead of being cured by giving them the right kind of food. Howard's theory, that food grown in humus is the

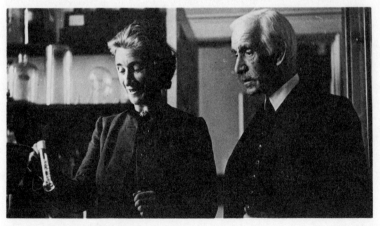

Sir Frederick Gowland Hopkins

only healthy kind, is as applicable to humans as to animals.

Lady Howard collaborated with her husband and propagated his idea after his death.

Hoxsey, Harry M, MD. Great-grandson of John Hoxsey, who in 1840 observed one of his horses which had contracted cancer, cure itself by selecting and eating certain herbs. He gathered these herbs, brewed them into a concoction and cured other cancerous animals. His knowledge was handed down to his son and grandson, and to his great-grandson when he was 18. Eventually he founded the Hoxsey Cancer Clinic in Dallas, Texas, where only herbal preparations were used. In 1953 Dr Martin Luis Guzman, Editor of the Mexican weekly *Tiempo* went to Dallas to investivate his claims and was told by doctors at the Clinic that 85% of external, and 25% internal, cases of cancer had been cured. In breast cancer the cures were 50-60%; and even cases of melanoma (black cancer), which according to the medical profession was fatal, had responded favourably to herbal medicine.

In 1924, under strict medical supervision, Hoxsey was permitted to try out his treatment on a 66-year-old sergeant of police, who was considered a terminal case with little chance of recovery, but under the Hoxsey treatment he recovered and a prominent medical leader announced to a group of assembled colleagues: 'Gentlemen, you have just witnessed the eighth wonder of the world! We have now a cure for cancer.' Instead of giving him every encouragement, however, the medical profession asked him to sign a contract making over to them his herbal formulae, and to deliver ten barrels of his internal medicines, and 100 lb of ointment; in addition he was to close his cancer clinic immediately and relinquish his practice. Further, the agreement stipulated, he would receive no reward for ten years, but after that period he would be given 10% of the net profits earned.

When Hoxsey refused to sign the contract he was threatened: 'If you treat another cancer case we'll send you to jail!' Hoxsey refused and continued his work, was hounded and persecuted, arrested four times for practising medicine without a licence, and on three occasions had to pay fines of 100 dollars. The American Medical Association, which is far more hide-bound than the BMA and guards its rights and privileges jealously, refused in spite of all evidence, to admit that Hoxsey had a cure for cancer and said that his formulae were worthless and 'little more than a cough mixture'. Some British researchers admit that herbs may cure cancer, but are reluctant to allow their names to be mentioned.

Humus. Vegetable mould; the dark-brown or black substance resulting from the slow decomposition of organic matter found beneath trees in woods and forests. This humus consists of decomposed leaves which fall each autumn, the droppings of insects birds and small animals and the moulds regurgitated by worms. Countless insects live in woods (2,000 species are said to inhabit the oak) and their bodies help to make humus. Unfortunately, it takes centuries to make one inch of humus on the forest floor, whereas Man can make humus, which he calls compost, from the skins and fruit of vegetables and fruit, garden waste, leaves, straw, grass, etc., with layers of earth between them and an activator to break down the lot. The mineral content of compost is increased if cow dung, horse, pig manure or chicken manure is added. This and grass generates heat and kills weeds, and compost properly made contains no weed seeds.

Professor Bottomley, the botanist, says that where soil bacteria is increased, the vitamins in plants are also increased, which is not the case when fertilisers are used. In Britain in 1970 small holdings produced 125,000,000 tons of excreta from cows, pigs, horses, chickens and sheep, but because of our policy of using artificials many farmers paid to get rid of it and £30,000,000 worth of fertiliser was imported. At that time a ton of poultry manure was worth £1.77, cow manure £0.66 and pig manure £0.61. If mixed with straw and spread on the land this would produce rich, health-giving compost.

Humus (and compost) has numerous other advantages over fertilisers: it holds moisture which enables crops to develop during periods of drought, attracts earth worms which enrich the soil and produces disease-resisting crops.

Hydrotherapy. From the Greek *hudor*, water, and *therapeutikos*, to take care of, to heal; the art of healing by water. Hydrotherapy in one or more of its various forms has been tried in different parts of the world for centuries. The Chinese, Hindus, Egyptians, Hebrews, Red Indians, Greeks and Romans practised the water-cure and within the last three centuries *Father Kneipp* in Germany and *Vincent Preissnitz* in Austria established spas that were famous. Later the cult came to Britain where Dr Gully founded the baths at Droitwich and Bath, to which the wealthy flocked to rid themselves of gout and other diseases brought about by gluttony and injudicious living.

Water treatment takes many forms: hot, cold and saline baths, hip baths (sitz baths), foot baths, hot-and-cold baths alternately, Turkish baths, sauna baths, the fry-and-freeze treatment of Dr St John Lyburn, and other varieties.

Turkish, sauna, friction and cold *sitz baths* are given to eliminate poisons; cold water packs to cure *rheumatism, constipation* and other diseases; to mend broken bones, relieve strains, and heal bruises and wounds. It is usual for hydrotherapy to be used in conjunction with *fasting,* herbal treatment and *food reform,* and apparent miracles have been achieved. The value of water both externally and internally cannot be over-emphasised; but haphazard treatment by the uninitiated can sometimes have disastrous results.

Hypnosis. From the Greek *hypnos,* sleep. A condition resembling sound sleep artificially induced, marked by subconscious activity and sensitivity to suggestion. Hypnosis is not true sleep in which the blood gradually drains from the brain causing brain anaemia, followed by loss of consciousness. During normal sleep it is impossible to perform the feats undertaken while under hypnosis; e.g. bear intolerable pain with impunity or recall incidents from the past that were forgotten. Dr Grey Walter says that whereas anaesthetics produce regular and striking changes in the brain rhythms and responses, hypnosis has no effect on them. 'Hypnosis,' he says, 'shows none of the electrical features of natural sleep; indeed, the more carefully we consider the subject's state, the less it seems to resemble anything we know of sleep. Awareness is not lost, but heightened – restricted, it is true, to certain categories of stimuli, usually the hypnotist's voice and suggestions.'

Under hypnosis the patient so responds that the chemistry of his blood may be changed, and a number of diseases which have defied orthodox treatment have responded to hypnotic suggestion, among them asthma and extreme cases of psoriasis. In Britain hypnosis, which originally was condemned by the BMA, is now a recognised form of therapy controlled by the Association of Medical Hypnotists.

Hypochondria. Derived from the Greek *hupo,* under, and *chonros,* a cartilage. An exaggerated or obsessive attention to, an anxiety about health. Most disease is *psychosomatic,* and hypochondriacs believe they are ill, or cause illness where none exists. They would do well to follow *Coue's* advice. See: Coue'.

I

Iodine. A non-metallic element found in minute quantities in many animals and plants. In its free state it is soluble in ether and alcohol, but imperfectly in water. It is present in the thyroid gland and is essential for the formation of an organic iodine compound – thyroxin – which regulates some of the metallic functions of the organism. A lack of iodine is responsible for the enlargement of the thyroid gland, or goitre. Goitre may also be caused by an unbalanced *diet,* or absence of iodine in the soil. As sea water contains iodine it is present in significant quantities in sea plants such as dulse, kelp, agar-agar, algae, etc. The French chemist Dr Bourcet, says that iodine is present in microscopic quantities in pineapple, green kidney beans, asparagus, cabbage, garlic, mushrooms, strawberries, whole rice, leeks, sorrel, green beans, tomatoes, pears, artichokes, dry white beans, lettuce, grapes, potatoes, oat flour, wholewheat flour and white flour. Iodine has numerous functions in the body, the most important being the metabolism of calcium and building resistance to harmful bacteria.

Ions. An electrically charged atom or group of atoms. Gaseous ions may be produced in gases by electric sparks, the passage of energetic charged particles, X-rays, gamma rays (q.v.), ultraviolet rays, etc. Ions in solution are caused by the ionisation of the dissolved substance. When water is sprayed from a fountain or a bathroom shower a field of negative electrification is created. The same action takes place in a waterfall or when rain falls just after a thunderstorm, especially after a long dry period. The air seems fresh, sweet and clean because it is charged with negative ions, which speed the delivery of oxygen to the tissues.

In 1967 the Russian scientist Igor Ostrayakov found during experiments that the right amount of negative ionisation speeds up plant growth, suppresses the development of fungus micro-organisms, improves the blood composition of animals and retards the growth of tumours. Inhaling high concentrations of negative ions also relieves hay fever and asthma. Doctors have found that ionization reduces pain in burns and the need for narcotics, and has had beneficial effects on cancer patients, but more research is needed before it can be said that the effect is permanent.

Iron. An essential constituent of the blood. The body of a man weighing 150 lb contains about one sixth of an ounce of iron. It is a catalyst and an oxidiser, and in humans and animals it is necessary for the process of respiration and is a part of haemoglobin, a protein containing pigment which in turn contains iron. Each molecule of haemoglobin contains four atoms of iron and each atom of iron combines with one molecule of oxygen. Most of it is stored in the liver where it is picked up by the blood and carried to the red marrow. Some of it goes into the bile and is excreted; that is why one needs some iron every day. The livers of animals, fish and birds contain most iron, but egg yolk and fresh vegetables also contain some. Lack of iron results in anaemia.

Iron is necessary for the assimilation of carbon dioxide and the synthesis of organic matter from inorganic matter in plants by means of chlorophyl and sunlight; for the process of respiration in all animals; for the generation of magnetic blood currents in the nerve spirals which pass through the walls of the arteries and veins. Most edibles contain traces of iron, the richest sources being liver, egg yolk, sorrel, lettuce, leeks, spinach, rice bran, strawberries, radishes, asparagus, onions, cabbage, pumpkin and cucumber.

Issels, Dr Joseph. A Swiss doctor who is said to have cured some cases of cancer by building up the body's resistance with improved *diet,* the removal of sources of infection such as bad teeth or inflamed tonsils, the stimulation of intestinal bacteria, the use of oxygen, ozone, drugs and artificially induced fever. Because his methods were unorthodox he was forced out of business in Germany, where he had a clinic and the medical profession barred him from giving interviews. In 1971, according to the *Sunday Times* (22.2.1976) a British medical team headed by Sir David Smithers, a leading radiotherapist, spent five days at his Ringberg Clinic in Bavaria and sharply criticised his methods. But many of his former patients were loyal to him, and 54-year-old George Chambers, who worked for British Rail, says he went to Dr Issels with an inoperable brain tumour, and 'He saved my life. I was a dead man when I went to see him. I have not had a check-up or any drugs for two years and I feel fine.' He is only one of many.

When his clinic was shut down Issels had debts amounting to £1,275,000 and was forced to sell his £300,000 home and other property. He has now opened on a small scale. Of the Smithers' Report, he says: 'The British medical group based its condemnation on only 45 cases and stayed only five days at the clinic to study 6,000 case histories.'

According to a biography on Issels, a number of British doctors did their utmost to prevent the BBC from making a documentary about his work entitled *Go Climb A Mountain*. It is true that Dr Issels tried to cure Lilian Board, the Olympic runner, but apparently she went to him when the disease, cancer, was in an advanced stage and she had been given up by the medical profession. When he failed to cure her he was condemned as a quack.

J

Jarvis, Dr D. C., MD. After qualifying as an ear, eye, nose and throat specialist, this fifth-generation Vermonter whose family and neighbours had practised folk-medicine, started to observe Nature and the ways of animals and birds and realised that instinctively they knew how to cure illness, and evolved his own system which included the eating of natural foods and herbs, to which he added *honey,* apple cider vinegar and seaweed. His fame rests mainly on his recommendation of apple cider vinegar for rheumatism, arthritis, obesity, chronic fatigue, headache, high blood pressure, dizziness, sore throat and a score of other complaints. His colleagues condemned his methods as 'unscientific' and articles by specialists in medical journals and magazines for the layman said his ideas were rubbish; but these were refuted by the tens of thousands he cured, who could find no relief at the hands of his orthodox colleagues. The writer owes him a debt for pointing out that *honeycomb* is a cure for hay fever. His books *Folk Medicine* and *Arthritis and Folk Medicine* have sold by the million.

Jogging. One of the latest crazes to sweep America, where comparatively few past the age of 40 play team games. They amble at a trot each morning and evening to cover a set distance. It is a mild form of running which helps to keep down the blood pressure and prevent hardening of the arteries, heart disease and osteo-arthritis. Constant gentle use of the limbs helps to prevent degenerative diseases, from which two people out of three over the age of 45 suffer. A survey carried out on 74 former athletes in Finland whose average age was 55, proved that joints are not worn out by constant use. Some of them had held world or national records and had competed, on average, for 21 years. Their hip joints and those of 115 non-athletes of similar age were compared and it was found that whereas only 4% of the athletes had osteo-arthritis, 8.7% of the non-athletes had the disease. It is now thought that the cartilage that lines the hip joint is nourished by a fluid which is released when the joint is moved. The more you use the joint, the more fluid is released. Immobility has the opposite effect and jogging is the answer. Jogging will be ineffective, however, if the *diet* is unbalanced.

Juices, Fruit. These contain, in small quantities, all the substances needed to nourish the body, but are not in any sense a substitute for food. Their value is intensified when ill, or fasting. Juices are highly concentrated and their action is powerful; the fit should dilute them generously with water and no more than half a wineglass of pure juice taken at a time. They are rich in minerals, act on the organs, glands and nervous system and are good for all kidney, bladder and digestive diseases, rheumatism, arthritis, etc.

K

K-Vitamin. See: Vitamin K.
Kellogg, John Harvey
(1855-1946) **FAMS, FRCS (Eng).**
A leading member of the
American Medical Association
and one of the most respected
vegetarians of his time who,
by his writing, books and
lectures helped to make
vegetarianism respectable in
America. Preached the gospel of
fresh air and sunshine and
invented several devices for the
administration of ultra-violet
and infra-red light. He stated that
'Medicine does not cure; only
Nature has the power to restore
the body.' He advocated simple

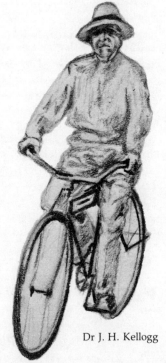

Dr J. H. Kellogg

food, mental hygiene, exercise and rest among pleasant surroundings. 'Hospitals,' he said, 'are places for the sick' and
founded a health home in Battle Creek which he called the
'Sanitarium'. When someone pointed out that there was no
such word, he retorted: 'But there soon will be.' The word is
now in *Webster's Dictionary*.

He declared that the mind is more important than the body
both in sickness and in health and encouraged convalescents to
walk, swim, play tennis and listen to music. He placed his
'visitors' (not patients) on a diet which excluded tea, coffee,
meats, condiments, highly seasoned foods and alcoholic drinks,
and waged a campaign against smoking. He cured so many
patients of TB that the AMA was enraged and declared him a
heretic. In spite of this the Kellogg Sanitarium grew famous and
was visited by celebrities such as Henry Ford, Billy Sunday,
Henry Firestone, Eva Booth, Lowell Thomas, Percy Grainger,
Tilden, Iturbi, Admiral Byrd, Amundssen, Adlai Stevenson,
Rockefeller, Franklin D. Roosevelt and others, who were made
to subsist on yogurt, molasses, honey, buttermilk, salads, fruit,
cheese, nuts and wholewheat bread. In time those who
regained health at the 'San' demanded the kind of food they
were given there, in their own homes, and the health-food
industry was started.

Kellogg, W. K. (1863-1958). Brother of J. H. Both were ardent
Seventh-day Adventists. By a process of trial and error Will
Kellogg produced shredded wheat, cornflakes, granola biscuits,
all-bran and other health foods such as protone, nutolene,
nut-wheat, etc., for those who had been 'visitors' at his
brother's Sanitarium. He also invented peanut butter which at
first was sold exclusively to Seventh-day Adventists. The
demand for health foods so increased that he built a factory to
produce them and advertised: WILL YOU LEAD THE BATTLE
CREEK LIFE FOR 30 DAYS? and offered customers a $4.50
assortment of health foods by mail, pointing out that health
foods needed no cooking. The flood of orders came so fast that
soon instead of selling 150 cases a day he had to build a station at
Battle Creek from which trains loaded with his foods left daily.

Within 20 years he was one of the richest men in America and
his company was spending 100,000,000 dollars a year on advertising alone. But Kellogg spent little on himself. He ate only two
meals a day; the first fruit juice, egg and cereal, and for dinner at
*American Medical Association

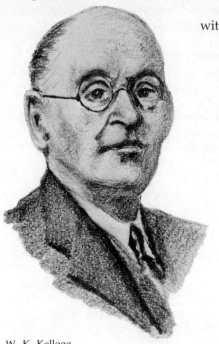

W. K. Kellogg

six, buttermilk sweetened with honey, salad with either potatoes in their jackets, or a cheese, egg or nut dish, followed by a sweet or savoury. Most of his millions went to finance his brother's enterprises or were ploughed back into the business. Both brothers invested money in educational trusts, hospitals and medical research, public health, dentistry, farming and agricultural schemes, and experiments; and for the alleviation of poverty in Africa, Asia and Europe. In 1930 the Kellogg Foundation was set up. It had an annual expenditure of more than 4,000,000 dollars on some 1,500 projects. J. H. had no hobbies or interests outside his work. W. K. was wiser. He took long holidays, combining business with pleasure, bought an 800-acre farm in Pomona, California, and reared some of the finest Arab thoroughbreds in the world. The ideas of the brothers, once considered revolutionary, are now held by millions.

King, Professor F. H. D.Sc. Professor of Agricultural Physics at the University of Wisconsin and Chief of the Division of Soil Management, US Department of Agriculture. He visited China and Japan where he studied the way in which these two peoples used every iota of human and animal wastes, together with leaves, straw, grass, etc., and turned it into compost to produce some of the healthiest crops in the world and feed a sturdy population free from the degenerative diseases of civilisation. He saw contractors bidding large sums for the privilege of carting away tons of human and animal wastes and selling them to farmers. Compared with the United States, where such wastes were poured into rivers and lakes, polluting them, and robbing the land of 12,000,000 lb of nitrogen each year, their system was enlightened and advanced. In China 150,000 tons of phosphorus, 376,000 tons of potassium, and 1,158,000 tons of nitrogen were put back into the soil. Dr King's book, *Farmers Of Forty Centuries,* which ran into many editions, is regarded as a classic and shows that the Chinese and Japanese were not only pioneers in this field but that no western nation is as yet as advanced in soil culture and, with few exceptions, we have learnt little from the lessons outlined in his book. He showed that if a nation is to be healthy and its husbandry efficient, everything that comes out of the soil must be replaced.

Kloss, Jethro (1863-1946). Born on a farm near Manittowac, Wisconsin, in primitive Indian country, Kloss learnt from the Indians, who knew the value of wild and cultivated herbs, grains, nuts, fruit and vegetables. His parents taught him to gather leaves, bark and berries and prepare infusions, poultices and healing unguents from them. Early in life he realised how disastrous was the use of drugs. In 1900 he married and operated a branch of the Battle Creek Sanitarium, and later, with his second wife, a pleasant health home called The Home Sanitarium which had a surgery attached where local surgeons performed operations while Kloss administered anaesthetics. He then branched out into the health-food business and set up factories for making his foods and cafeterias and schools where he disposed of his products. Kloss cured every disease in the medical encyclopaedia without resorting to drugs: asthma, rheumatism, arthritis, tuberculosis (then considered incurable), diabetes, paralysis and even cancer if these were taken in hand in time. He fasted patients and prescribed herbs, *hydrotherapy* and *food reform.* He wore himself out in the service of suffering humanity but fortunately, much of the knowledge he acquired is condensed in *Back to Eden,* one of the best books of its kind.

Kneipp, Father Sebastian (1821-1897). Kneipp is generally regarded as the great 'water doctor', but he was a thinker who unearthed and used a number of natural methods of healing. He drew attention to the healing power of plants and made medicines from them. Kneipp believed in the *whole* power of plants: roots, bark, stem, leaves and flowers, in their natural state and refused to administer extracts. He used infusions, decoctions and tinctures, and herbs in cooking. In *So Sollt Ihr Leben* (Thus Thou Shalt Live) he argued for a return to Nature and coarse home-woven shirts and under pants. Clothes should

79

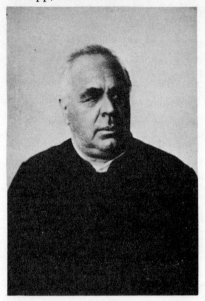

Father Sebastian Kneipp

be soft, light and not too tightly woven; people should live outdoors most of the day and not in over-heated rooms. He founded *Kinderaysl* (homes for poor children) in Worishofen, where they could live in harmony with Nature. He also maintained that his methods would have no permanent value unless endorsed by the medical fraternity and was so successful that doctors from all over the world made their way to Bavaria to learn his methods. Kneipp started life with few advantages for he was the son of a weaver in Stefansried, whose wife and children had to share his work. He worked as a farmer's boy in summer and a weaver in winter. His ambition was to become a Catholic priest and he found a protector in the village chaplain Mathias Merkle, who prepared him for the grammer school, after which he studied theology in Dillingen and Munich. But excessive work and privations undermined his health, he developed tuberculosis and was given up by doctors. Then a friend in the State Library gave him a book on water treatment by Hahn and Kneipp followed his teachings. Several times a week, after dark, he ran to the Danube, half an hour away, and plunged into its icy depths; then dressed rapidly and returned home at a brisk trot. This drastic treatment made him feel better each time, till eventually after months he was completely cured. Then he turned his attentions to a student with the same disease and cured him. After which he was appointed father confessor to the Dominican nuns at Worishofen, where he cured the sick with water. One of his first cures was that of a woman with varicose veins and festering sores on her legs, which had defied the efforts of the local physician, who was much impressed when he observed the result.

Kneipp's fame grew so rapidly that Pope Leo XIII who was ill, sent for him, followed his instructions and regained health. His water treatment was not drastic; the colder the water, the shorter the time of immersion. He also used compresses, massage and exercise, and all his patients were kept on a diet of fruit, vegetables, nuts, herbal tissanes, and given plenty of fresh air.

He treated more than 100,000 patients, lectured widely and wrote a number of books that were read avidly by the *Naturarzt* (natural healing) fraternity. His advice is still followed at the clinic he founded in Worishofen.

L

Laughter. One of the finest tonics on earth which, in the music hall in Victorian England often made the lives of the very poor bearable, for they looked forward to visiting the theatre on Saturday nights. If you have a sense of humour which enables you to laugh not only at others but at yourself, nothing will get you down. Jews, for instance, a race depressed and persecuted for centuries, have a wonderful sense of humour and a fund of jokes against themselves, one reason for their resiliance and excellent health. Negroes, too, whether Africans or West Indians, bubble with good humour, laughter and song which enables them to rise above the most squalid conditions.

Hearty laughter is a tonic which dissipates gloom, gets rid of inhibitions and exercises the stomach muscles and the diaphragm. To be rendered 'weak with laughter' is a good thing. Dr Pierre Vachet, a famous Parisian, used to give practical lessons in the art of laughter every Sunday morning to an assembly of people of all ages and from all walks of life. He used to start by saying: 'My friends, you have come here to laugh, to bathe in an atmosphere of happiness that will restore your health and spirits. We have within us emotional forces which can be released by laughter.' He would then instruct them to close their eyes, sit comfortably and put their minds to sleep. When the room was quiet a gramophone record exclusively of laughter would be played – laughter of every kind – till gradually his audience became infected and laughter resounded through the auditorium. It gained in volume till everyone was shaking with laughter. Then Vachet would command: 'Lights!' and everywhere one would see relaxed happy faces.

'Laughter,' he said, 'releases tonic emotions which through the medium of the sympathetic nervous system cause a sudden nervous discharge and change the physiological reactions of the individual.'

At New York University an experiment was carried out with two groups of students. One was given scientific discussions after meals; the other was entertained by comedians. After only two weeks it was found that the spirits, digestion and general health of the second group had improved noticeably.

Rebelais, who was a doctor, advised: 'Burst with laughter and get well.' The man (or woman) with pursed lips and a constant look of disapproval, who regards a joke as an obscenity, usually has something wrong with his health and more often than not with his digestion. See: Emotions, Fears.

Leeches. See: Venesection.

Legumes *(Leguminosae).* A family which includes peas, beans and pulses. Leguminous plants are cultivated in many parts of the world. The common pea *(pisum sativum)* and the *lentil* have been grown for centuries around the Mediterranean coasts, Asia and America, where the Lima bean, kidney, haricot and French bean also flourish. The soya bean *(Glycine max)* and the ground pea *(Arachis hypogaea)* are grown in China and Brazil. Legumes, mentioned in the Bible, have been eaten all over Asia Minor and the East for centuries and when the Romans conquered Britain they introduced the lentil because it was easily carried, did not deteriorate, and as a food was both nourishing and sustaining. Legumes are valued for their high protein content and comparatively low cost. See: Lentils.

Lemon. Valued since the seventeenth century for its anti-scorbutic properties. In 1753 James Lind wrote *A Treatise On Scurvy,* a comprehensive study of the disease, in which he recommended lemons as a cure. An analysis of the lemon shows that it has the highest vitamin C content of all citrus fruits: 1,200 IU per 100 grammes. Regular intake of the juice maintains the vitamin C content of the

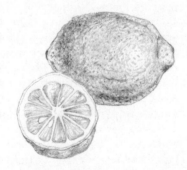

body, helps to ward off colds and influenza, and is of value during fasts.

Lentils. Known as 'Poor Man's Meat' in India and Pakistan. Till recently it was used in Britain only to make dishes such as pease pudding but the influx of Indian and Pakistani immigrants with new and exotic dishes, both savoury and sweet, made from lentils, has introduced a new chapter into British cuisine. There are various kinds of lentils: red, yellow, black and white. They contain 25.70% of protein (beef has only 20.00%) but are not easily digested for they are rich in fat and contain other substances antagonistic to digestion. No more than 2 oz of lentils a day should be eaten though a person with a sound digestion can handle 3 oz, and labourers engaged in heavy work have been known to consume 8 oz. About 2½ oz (70 grammes) are sufficient if no other form of protein is eaten, and the average person can live on lentils as the main form of protein, without touching meat. Indeed, millions in Africa and the East do so. Lentils should always be put into boiling water and then simmered because if the water is cold and then brought to the boil they do not break down easily. They are a valuable food for all on a strictly limited budget. See: Legumes

Leyel, Mrs F. C. Though in the past herbalism flourished in Britain, it fell into disrepute, and its present popularity is due largely to Mrs Leyel and her many books on the subject: *Herbal Delights, Compassionate Herbs, Green Medicine, Elixirs of Life, Hearts-Ease, Cinquefoil,* etc. She started her work as a firm believer in orthodox medicine, devoting years to collecting money for medical institutions and hospitals – nearly £1,000,000. For her labours she was made a life governor of St Mary's Hospital, The Royal National Orthopaedic Hospital, and the West London Hospital. She also made a study of herbs and felt that they were not used as widely or as effectively as they should be and, influenced by the work of *Hahnemann,* devoted her life to herbalism. Originally the word drug meant any complete medicinal plant or crude substance used as a medicine; but today 'drug' is usually taken to mean a refined derivative, which is the result of the modern pharmaceutical practice of extracting from a plant its alkaloids or active principles, and discarding every other element of which the plant is composed, so changing it from an organic into an inorganic substance. It became her purpose in life to rectify this and she cured thousands who medical science failed to cure, and founded the House of Culpepper, named after the most famous of British herbalists. There are other herbalists perhaps more knowledgeable, whose businesses have flourished for more than 100 years, but they lacked her flair and she, more than anyone, has been instrumental in rehabilitating the science of *herbalism*. See: Herbalism.

Lief, Peter. Born in 1927 the son of Stanley Lief (which see) he was reared on health reform lines which continued even while a pupil at boarding school. Volunteered for the Royal Navy in 1943, was exempt from vaccination and immunisation when sent to the Far East but remained immune to cholera, malaria, typhoid and other tropical diseases to which many other ratings succumbed. Though by no means robust he represented both his school and naval unit at rugby, tennis and swimming. After the war he entered Northwestern University and then the Osteopathic College in Chicago and within three years was transformed from an eight-stone weakling into a 13½ stone wrestler. He worked at Champneys the well-known health home owned and run by his father. When Stanley Lief retired Peter moved to London and set up in practice. For a time, until pressure of work made him relinquish the job, he was Editor of the magazine *Health For All,* founded by his father, and now he is in full time practice at Enton Hall.

Leif, Stanley (1892-1963). Born in Russia, one of a family of eight children. His father, a soldier in the pay of the Czar, was poor, so the family fled to South Africa and settled in Pretoria where Lief spent a boyhood ridden by illness. He was too fat and had a weak heart. Doctors could do little for him; as a result he grew shy and introspective, helped his father in his grocery store and studied engineering. Often he sat watching the Africans at work and observed that when they were sick they just lay in

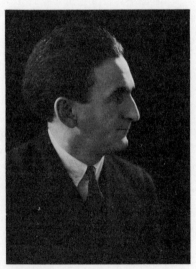

Stanley Lief

the sun and refused to eat till well again. He became so interested in this 'instinctive fasting' that he decided to copy them and his health improved vastly. Wishing to learn more, he searched the bookstalls and came across *Bernarr Macfadden's Physical Culture* magazine. After devouring a number of issues he was so inspired that he informed his parents of his wish to devote his life to natural healing, and was ridiculed.

At 18 he left home and worked his way to America as a ship's steward, went to Chicago and enrolled in the Macfadden college, where he emerged as their star student, built up his physique and became wrestling champion of Illinois. Then he travelled the States, widening his knowledge at various health establishments and eventually sailed for Britain where he helped to run the Macfadden Health Home in Brighton. He volunteered during the 1914 war, was made a physical culture instructor, went to France and in 1918 was invalided out of the army with a shrapnel wound in one arm, which the surgeons told him would have to be amputated. He refused to accept their verdict and for six months lived according to vegetarian principles, fasted occasionally, dressed his own wounds, exercised and regained the full use and mobility of his arm.

He then went to Bristol where he eked out a living by writing health articles and working as a masseur in a health home. From then his progress was phenomenal and within a year he bought out the owner. At first all his patients were men and women who had been pronounced 'incurables' by the medical profession but he cured most of them. Patients flocked to him and in 1925, with the help of C. M. Trelawney-Irving, a grateful patient (he died well over 90) he bought Champneys, which until his death was Britain's best known health home. Many of the famous went there to regain their health. *Health For All* was founded by him in 1927; it was by far the best health magazine in the country till it ceased publication in 1967.

Light. Dr Rollier of Leysin, one of the pioneers of light therapy, regarded the *skin* as the most important organ in the body and said that if deprived of light it would not function normally. Natural light prevents wasting of the muscles. Sir Henry Gauvin, a British pioneer, was convinced that light is needed for brain development. Both Arnold Rikli and J. P. Muller advocated the full exposure of the naked body to light and air. In 1928 Dame Kathleen Olga Vaughan, MB (Lond), who had worked among the women of Kashmir came to the same conclusion.

Many of the women suffered from osteomalacia because they worked in deep valleys clothed in mist and lived in homes where the windows were usually cemented into place, and the glass cut off all ultra-violet rays below 330 mm. These and other findings show that light – not merely sunlight – is important to health and if deprived of it, or if the light is always filtered through glass, health invariably suffers.

Lime. Fruit of the citrus family akin to lemon, which has a green rind and a much pleasanter aroma and flavour than the lemon, though it contains less *vitamin C*. Lime juice contains 750 IU per 100 grammes. Its lack of acidity adds to its value, for whereas limes are usually eaten, lemons rarely are.

Lind, James. See: Lemon.

Lindlhar, Henry, MD. Before the First World War *Nature Cure* was taught in a somewhat haphazard way but towards the end of the war Lindlhar established his College of Natural Therapeutics where he harmonised the many strands of the movement and organised it till it had a large following. He maintained that most diseases were caused by the wrong emotions to which all are at times subject but that there was no such thing as a cure-all; 'if there were, it would be cold water, properly applied.' He successfully treated thousands of patients, using only the simplest equipment, such as was to be found in the home of every peasant. His principle was that in all treatments the patient's reactions must be observed and act as a guide, especially in the use of cold water, for all do not react in the same way. Water treatment is extremely effective if applied according to his instructions and there is no need for any patient to be unduly spartan. His *Practice of Nature Cure* is as true today as when it was written.

He insisted that health lay in the soil and that all wastes should be returned to it. 'In our institution,' he said; 'we begin the treatment of patients by treating the soil of our gardens and farmlands with mineral fertilisers. For many seasons now we have saturated the land with wood ash, sifted coal finely pulverised lime rock, pulverised phosphate rock and iron filings with small quantities of rock-salt. The effect of this continued, systematic, mineral fertilising on the products of our gardens has been little short of marvellous. It is natural that the manufacturers of the usual commercial fertilisers, containing a surplus of nitrogen and phosphates, strenuously oppose all new ideas of sensible soil culture and condemn all mineral fertilisers as worthless and fraudulent.'

Ling, Per Hendrik (1776-1839). Born near Reashult, Sweden and known as the Father of European Physical Culture. He was opposed to brute force and his system of gymnastics was designed to increase suppleness, speed, agility and strength; make one breathe more deeply, and cause the flow of blood to increase and so help to cure diseases. He founded the first gymnasium in Stockholm in 1813, built the first swimming pool in Europe (people had hitherto swum in Lakes, rivers and the sea), and laid emphasis on the value of games and sport. He deplored specialisation, advocated moderation in all things and warned against over-exercise.

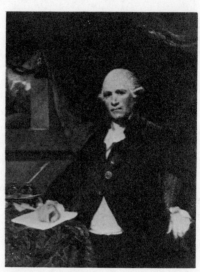

Per Henrik Ling

He reduced the obese, cured abnormalities such as kyphosis (round back), lordosis (hollow back), and flat feet, and his system cured many people of lung trouble.

Ling institutes flourished in Sweden and today there are hundreds all over the world, with 4,000 Ling Associates in Britain where it is popular because it is rhythmic without a jerky movement in any of its exercises.

Liquorice (Glycorrizha glabra). Known to the public in Britain mainly as a base for sweets such as 'liquorice all-sorts', Pontefract cakes, Spanish ribbons and Spanish sticks, but in the past Moorish physicians gave it to women who could not conceive and for more than 2,000 years it has been used for coughs and chest complaints by herbalists as it is a demulcent, an emolient and an expectorant. Pure liquorice is made by boiling the roots of *glycorrizha glabra* into a thick syrup which coagulates when cooked, and when manufactured into sweets and unpleasant tasting drugs it is mixed with sugar. In 1946 its properties were investigated by a Dutch physician who found that some patients suffering from ulcers obtained lasting relief when a liquorice-based remedy made up by a local chemist in Heerenveen was taken; and recent German research indicates that it may be a safer remedy for rheumatic sufferers than cortisone.

Locke, Dr Mahlon W., MD. Celebrated as the 'foot-twister' of Williamsburg, Ontario, and ironically by the AMA* as the 'Miracle man of 1932'. He claimed to cure more people than any doctor in the world – more even than some large hospitals! For years he averaged 600 patients a day, charging each one dollar; no more, no less, making £30,000 a year. His surgery, a room in a farmhouse, was equipped with a table on which his patients lay. 'There is nothing magical about my treatment,' he said, 'the main nerve of each leg runs through the arch of the foot. There are four bones in this arch. If the arch falls the bones are thrown out of alignment, resulting in a pressure on the nerve. When the nerve is mashed between the joints of the arch, pain results, but not necessarily at that point. Pain in many parts of the body, called 'referred pain,' breaks out, setting up disturbances all over the body. One consequence is arthritis, while often muscular atrophy and certain forms of paralysis result.

'I simply thrust the arch of the foot back into its proper alignment, and the body, when relieved of pain, fights the germs for itself, thus aiding the cure of many diseases caused by germs.'

This explanation was not 'scientific' enough to satisfy the AMA but they were helpless to strike him off the register as he broke no rules. Patients whom doctors had failed to cure, flocked to him from every state in America, from Canada and from abroad. They limped to him, some on crutches and others on beds; the cars they came in formed a mile-long queue. Hotels and restaurants were built to cater for his 'pilgrims', who departed leaving behind sticks, crutches and bath chairs. He was the oddest practitioner in the American continent.

*American Medical Association.

Love. Affection, tenderness and the knowledge that you are appreciated and will be missed if absent, are potent factors in health. This is not always realised, especially in institutions where orphans, deprived children and those separated from parents, are kept. Lack of love affects not only the mentality but the chemistry of the blood. One of the first experiments proving this was carried out at the command of the Emperor Frederick II of Germany in the thirteenth century, who wanted to know what language a child would speak if untaught: Hebrew, Greek or its native tongue. A number of new-born orphans were placed in the charge of nurses who were instructed to provide them with every necessity, but neither to speak to them nor give them any signs of affection. All the infants died within months because they could not live without the facial expressions, cooing talk, hugs and kisses that mothers bestow on their babies.

This, according to Professor Eric Stroud, in charge of Child Health at King's College Hospital, London, applies in all phases of life; between parents and children, husbands and wives, brothers and sisters. Lack of affection and appreciation can be disastrous and is the cause of much introversion. There are numerous cases of lonely people committing suicide because they were unloved, and one who tried to poison her entire family as an act of revenge, told the judge when she was prosecuted: 'I did it because no one loves me.'

One reason why the children of large, poor families grow up strong and healthy, is that there exists a strong bond of love between them all. They care for, and try to help, each other. Love sustains, whereas indifference can destroy. See: Emotions, Tears, Laughter.

M

McCann, Alfred W. Before the First World War McCann was advertising manager of a food factory with a turnover of 12,000,000 dollars a year and for five years before the war he worked in the laboratory. He became convinced that no food reform can come through advertising. 'The advertising manager,' he declared, 'cannot state the whole truth in a food advertising campaign for the reason that manufacturers insist that advertisements shall center about the talking points that sell their products, always keeping clear of controversy.' He became so dissatisfied that *The Globe,* a New York paper equipped a laboratory and gave him freedom to report the results of his findings without regard to their influence on their advertising revenue. Soon 41 other periodicals in as many states took up his work but so severe was the pressure from advertising agencies that all, with the exception of *Chicago Daily News* discontinued their exposures.

During his period with *The Globe* he was made Deputy Health Commissioner by five New York municipalities and was employed by many mayors and police commissioners to make surveys of food conditions in their areas. He led squads of plain clothes men and trained agents, including attorneys and physicians, on raids that resulted in scores of indictments, trials and convictions. He was used by the US Department of Justice, the Attorney-General of New York State and by numerous public prosecutors, and was involved in 206 successful prosecutions. He never lost a case. His evidence about processing, denaturing, the colouring of food, etc., is given in *The Science of Eating,* which after the war made millions of Americans health-food conscious.

His most dramatic success occurred when the 'Kronprinz Wilhelm', a converted German cruiser which had sunk 14 ships and transferred their cargoes to his vessel, was forced to put into Newport Mews because 110 of her crew were prostrate with beri-beri and many more were down with various stages of the disease. The captain sought the help of American medical specialists, but they could do nothing. Eventually by a subterfuge, McCann made his way aboard, confronted the Chief Surgeon and told him he could cure the stricken men. The ship's hold was crammed with contraband: meat, butter, white flour, tea, biscuits, sweets, canned vegetables, sugar, etc., which McCann said was useless dead food.

He ordered that the sick men were to be fed on fresh vegetables and fruit, and that 200 lb of wheat *bran* be soaked in water at 120°F for twelve hours, then drained and each man be given 8 oz of the liquid each morning. In addition hundreds of pounds of potatoes were peeled, the *potatoes* discarded and the skins boiled. Each man was given 4 oz of the liquor each day. They were also given the diluted juice of ripe *oranges* and *lemons.*

Within five days no new cases of the disease were reported; within six, the symptons started to disappear; and in ten days 14 men were able to leave the ship's hospital. Dr Perronon, the

Chief Surgeon, reported that all the men were responding to treatment and one, who was completely paralysed, could stand without aid. Eventually all recovered. After McCann gave Surgeon-General Blue of the US Army the results of the case, he turned it over to the authorities, who suppressed the entire account and the benefits of the experiments were lost to the public for some years, till McCann's book was published.

McCarrison, Major-General, Sir Robert, CIE, MA, DSc, LLD, FRCP. Formerly Director of Research on Nutrition in India. India was his laboratory and with his original mind he made a major contribution to the science of nutrition. In 1936 he published his Cantor Lectures under the title *Nutrition and National Health* which was recognised throughout the world as the key work on the relation between properly constituted food and sound health. Unlike the peoples of most countries the Indian races differ widely in the food they eat and their physiques. He was among the first to correlate the two by studying the physiques of the Hunzas, whom he called the most perfect physical specimens in the world, and comparing them with other races in the sub-continent: Sikhs, Tibetan hillmen, Nepalese, Mahrattas, Pathans, Madrassis and Bengalis.

The Hunzas live in the Himalayas and their diet was derived mainly from vegetable sources, milk products and meat about once a month. The diet of the Bengalis and Madrassis was largely vegetable with very little protein; and the Bengalis lived mainly on fruit and vegetables, milk and fish with about 50 gm of protein a day. The Madrassis ate no animal protein; and these two races had the poorest physiques.

The Hunzas were by far the fittest of all groups and disease was virtually unknown among them. Their bodies were so tough that they plunged into mountain pools and enjoyed swimming in the icy waters. Their teeth were perfect and they died only when their bodies wore out. Since McCarrison's day they have been introduced to white flour products, white sugar, biscuits and refined foods, and as a result their general health has deteriorated. McCarrison found that among the Hunzas the degenerative diseases of civilisation, such as stomach ulcers, divertiliculitis, appendicitis, etc., were unknown. His research did more than anything to awaken the nations of the world to the dangers of malnutrition because of the lack of essential elements in food, and he stressed the point that fruit, vegetables and whole foods are best.

MacFadden, Bernarr. Pioneer of healthy living in the United States, whose ideas and teachings have spread to every continent and changed our conception of healthy living. He was a vegetarian, a sensationalist and a crank of the worst type. He had to be, to get his message home for he had to fight against ignorance, prejudice and commercial interests. He preached the doctrine of a *vegetarian diet, fasting,* fresh air, *exercise, hydrotherapy* and *nudism* to a Victorian society and achieved results by shocking the public. Like all iconoclasts he was a tyrant who believed that his ideas were right, the only ones worth having, and those who differed were wrong.

He was a wrestling champion and put his ideas before the public in a magazine he founded called *Physical Culture*. When he married a perfect physical specimen and produced seven lovely daughters he forced them to adopt his strict regimen, making them eat raw carrots, exercise with dumb-bells, bathe in cold water, winter and summer, and walk bare-foot on dewy grass. At one period he used to rise at four in the morning and walk 13 miles, bare-foot, to his office in New York. He never wore a collar or tie. His principles, and the health home he started made him famous and hundreds from every state in the Union flocked to learn about his methods and practise them. Later he founded the Macfadden Trust for the propagation of his ideas and was the first man to speak and write openly about the evils of venereal disease. For this he was prosecuted and sentenced to two years in prison but the outcry by senators, ministers of the churches and prominent public men was so great that President Taft had it rescinded two days later, and Macfadden launched a crusade to wipe out VD.

The ballyhoo was necessary for, in the main, what he advocated was sound. His doctrine is as true today as it was then and, making allowances for his extremism, he was in a sense a great man. No pioneer of vegetarianism has ever made such an impact on the world and though he was the *ne plus ultra* of all cranks he did an enormous amount of good. Many of the campaigns he started – good soil, whole foods, *exercise, hydrotherapy,* fresh air, etc. – are still being fought.

Macrobiotics. This is not as so many imagine, a diet exclusively of cooked vegetables and brown rice, but the principle of choosing food based on common sense, originated by Georges Ohsawa (1893-1966) and based on the Chinese system of Yang and Yin, which represent the positive and negative life forces. Every article of diet is either predominantly yang or yin and there is no single macrobiotic diet for every person. Consumption of the staple foods of the region in which one lives, is the right principle: oats and herrings, for instance, for the Scots; rice and fish for the Bengali; meat and blubber for the Eskimo; vegetables and sea food for the Japanese; spaghetti, olive oil and tomatoes for Italians.

Today with the interchange of ideas and foods few live on their ancient traditional diets but according to macrobiotics whole grains are common to all: wheat, corn, oats, barley, rye, millet, buckwheat, etc., should comprise the main part of every meal, for they are 'live', plentiful and economical. Refined grains should not be eaten.

Secondary foods consist of fresh vegetables, excluding potatoes and tomatoes; sea vegetables, beans, legumes and seeds. Soya beans are high-grade protein.

Other foods should be eaten occasionally, such as fresh fruit, dried fruit, raw vegetables, nuts, fish and occasionally, animal products.

Sweets should be from natural sources. Honey may be used occasionally, but neither brown nor refined sugars; and seasoning, only if it combines flavour with some nutritional value.

The only beverages allowed are green and twig teas and coffee made from roasted grains, beans and the roots of the dandelion or burdock. Liquids should be severely curtailed.

Before meals the emotional condition should be observed and foods that cause harmful emotions excluded. In cold climates the foods should be predominantly yang: fish, eggs, buckwheat, rice and vegetables; in torrid zones more yin: rice, wheat, oats, salads, honey, raw vegetables and fruit. For heavy labour, more yang foods than yin are needed.

Followers of macrobiotics are urged to avoid being dogmatic; to experiment, observe and learn from mistakes. The system is aimed to bring one into harmony with Nature and develop an appreciation of the simple things in life.

Magnesium. The body of a man weighing 150 lb contains about 1½ oz of magnesium, an acid-binding element, which exists in the body principally as phosphate of magnesia in the bones. These contain about 50% phosphate of lime and one per cent phosphate of magnesia. This small quantity gives the skeleton its firmness and prevents softening of the bones. Magnesium, together with *calcium, iron* and *sulphur* are involved in forming the albumen of the blood. Healthy lungs show twice as much magnesium as lime; and salts of magnesium are cell builders, particularly of lung tissue and the nervous system. Magnesium salts can perform their functions only if calcium salts are present, and their presence is necessary in healthy soil. In the body magnesium has particular vitalising powers.

Mango. The king of South-East Asian fruits. It was cultivated in India since time immemorial, is mentioned in ancient Sanskrit literature, and praised by Amir Krusru, the famous Turkoman poet. Akbar the Moghul emperor so prized the mango that he 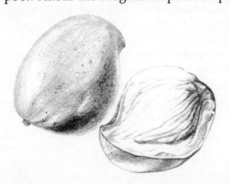 planted 100,000 mango trees at Lal Bagh, his famous orchard near Darbhanga. Today it is grown in South China, the Malay archipelago, Madagascar, tropical Africa, Burma, Egypt, Persia, Brazil, the West Indies and the USA. In India there are 500 varieties. The flavour of the best varieties is delicious and they are rich in fruit sugar. The unripe mango, used for making jam, chutney and pickle, contains tartaric, malic and a trace of citric acid, and 4,800 IU of vitamin A per 100 grammes. There is no fruit to compare with it and the Ayurveda recommends the eating of mangoes for growth, longevity and defective vision. It is also a good source of *niacin, riboflavin,* and its *vitamin C* content is four times that of the apple. It is laxative if eaten in sufficient quantity, has long been recommended for liver disorders and is excellent for convalescents and all who wish to put on weight. Delicious sherbets are made from mangoes, milk and ice. It contains 87.40% water, 0.06% protein, 0.40% fat, 9.90% carbohydrates and 0.50% mineral matter, mainly *potassium.*

Massage. In all ancient civilisations kneading and stroking the limbs, back, chest and neck has been carried out on the suffering to relieve pain. The Greeks and Romans were believers in the efficacy of massage and friction was practised by the Greeks 3,000 years ago. In the fifth century BC Hippocrates said it was a valuable pain reliever; it was used to relax patients and to mobilise unstable* and stiff joints. Galen wrote four treatises in the third century AD on active and passive massage and in Egypt and India the system never fell into disuse as it seems to have done in Europe. It was revived in the nineteenth century in Sweden, France and Britain and in 1836 Maignein reported excellent results in treating sprains.

Massage (1) rids the muscles of waste substances which accumulate in them and cause stiffness, fatigue and pain (2) it produces additional growth of bone and muscle and (3) has an important effect on the nervous system. Massage may take the form of rubbing, friction, kneading or vibration and all these movements increase circulation in the blood vessels in the parts massaged. An increase also takes place in the production of heat, which results in an increase in lung and muscle respiration. Limbs constantly massaged in the right way retain their youthful appearance far longer than those that are not. There are many variations of massage: (a) stroking (b) deep stroking (c) kneading (d) tapping and knocking (e) slapping (f) hacking and sawing (g) pressing, pushing and vibrating. The best results are produced when it is done in conjunction with calisthenics, hot and cold baths and packs, constant fresh air and a balanced diet.

Maxalding. A system of body building by means of muscle control named after Max Sick, an Austrian strong man in the early 1920s. Some of the exercises were based on the *bandhas* and *mudras* which are part of *hatha-yoga* philosophy, and lead to the awakening of *kundalini*. Max Sick used to have his chest bound in chains, which he snapped by flexing his muscles through mind control. The yogis have maintained for 6,000 years that mental control develops muscles more supple, flexible and of a higher quality than those developed merely by weights and other forms of resistance. The Maxalding system, still used by strong men who give exhibitions of muscle control on TV and the stage, is useful in the cure of constipation for it strengthens the diaphragm and the abdominal muscles.

Mazdaznan Science Of Right Living. A philosophy which includes rhythmic breathing, glandular therapy, personal diagnosis and higher eugenics, and a belief in the message of the pyramids. The Mazdaznan Science of Right Living was first expounded by Dr Otoman Zar-Adusht Ha'nish. Each meeting opens with rhythmic exercises followed by the serving of herb tea. The leader is known as Guromano, meaning Wise Man, and women leaders are known as Mothers. During the singing of hymns the congregation sits, performing exercises. A mirror is passed round into which each member gazes. It is then considered holy as each one has projected himself (or herself) into it. Past members included Henry Ford, Edison, President Masaryk of Czechoslovakia, and Hitler.

Meat. Meat is not now used in the biblical sense, or as the edible part of fruit, nuts, eggs, etc.; as in Shakespeare: 'Thy head is full of quarrels, as an egg is full of meat.' Today meat usually means flesh or sea foods. No one except a crank or a bigot will condemn meat-eating out of hand for millions of meat-eaters live long and healthy lives and some become centenarians.

There are excellent reasons for abstaining from flesh foods but few *vegetarians* put these forward. Excess of meat, or even meat-eating for many years, tends to undermine the internal organs, and Pavlov showed that the liver has three times as much work to do on a meat diet as on a vegetarian one. The idea that meat increases endurance is also erroneous for Dr Fish and Dr Fisher say in their book *How To Live:* 'Meat-eating and a high *protein* diet, instead of increasing endurance, have shown that, like alcohol, it actually reduces it;' and a *Report Of The United States National Conservation Commission* (Vol. III, p. 665) states: 'Comparative experiments on 17 vegetarians and 25 meat-eaters in the laboratory of the University of Brussels have shown little difference in strength between the two classes, but a marked superiority of the vegetarians in point of endurance.'

As we grow older the body deteriorates and the digestive and eliminative organs are less able to cope with flesh foods than those of vegetable origin. After 40 or 50 the wise eater will cut down on flesh products, especially those abundant in fat, such as pork, fatty meat and herrings and fried foods, of whatever origin. Many meat-eaters have turned to an entirely lacto-vegetarian diet after middle age, with excellent results. A meat meal should always be accompanied or followed by a fresh salad, for meat is *acid*-forming and fresh fruit and green, leafy vegetables are *alkaline*-forming, and a correct balance, essential to health, will be maintained. See: Vegetarianism.

Mellanby, Sir Edward (1884-1955). Distinguished physician and authority on nutrition, whose contribution to medical science included the discovery of *vitamin D* and the work leading to its separation from *vitamin A*, which were once thought to be the same. Born in Hartlepool, educated at Barnard Castle School and Cambridge University. After two years' research at

Emmanuel College he entered St. Thomas's Hospital. In 1910 he lectured on, and was Professor of, Philosophy at King's College, London. After doing further research at Cambridge, he was appointed to the chair of Pharmacology at Sheffield University.

While in London he worked on *vitamin* research under Gowland Hopkins, with a special interest in the causation of rickets, and found that this disease could be prevented by a substance soluble in fat – fish or animal – but not in vegetable oils. It was abundant in fish oils, especially cod liver. He and his colleagues eventually separated vitamin D from A.

Later Mellanby proved that a lack of vitamin A often produced deep neurological disorders because of the mechanical effect of abnormal bone growth around the foramina through which the nerves leave the central nervous system. He also studied the effects of agene, used in bleaching white bread (which caused hysteria in dogs), and the effects on health where *iodine* was lacking, as a cause of goitre. Between 1933-1949 Mellanby was Secretary of the Medical Research Council.

Melon. A name for several kinds of gourd bearing sweet tropical fruit with thirst quenching properties. Melons contain a great deal of water, have a very low calorific value and contain vitamins A and C. As they are sweet, sugar should not be sprinkled on them. Some varieties are astringent, and they are strongly alkaline.

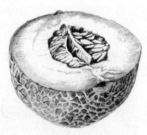

Mesmer, Franciscus Antonius (1733-1815). Born in Iznag, Germany and educated at the Jesuit College, Dillingen. He grew more interested in science than theology, forsook the Church and enrolled in the medical school of the University of Vienna. Financially independent, he was able to experiment and put many of his theories into practice. He wrote a book entitled *De Platinarium Influx* in which he explained that a mysterious fluid emanated from the stars, filling the universe and, if a proper balance was not maintained between this fluid and the body, disease would result. He used to 'magnetise' bits of wood and glasses of water and patients who touched the wood and drank the water were cured of their ills. It was believed that neither wood nor water can be magnetised, but when Mesmer, robed

97

impressively, walked among his patients and passed his hands over them while soft music was played behind thick curtains, he mesmerised them. He used suggestion to cure and explained that a healing fluid emanated from the brain, nerves and will, which he called 'animal magnetism.' This was nothing less than hypnotic suggestion, originally called mesmerism, after him.

Though he was hounded by the medical profession the King of Prussia sent Wolfat, his personal physician, to study under Mesmer, and the Russian and Austrian governments also sent their experts to learn his methods. He journeyed to Paris where Marie Antoinette became his patron. During the Revolution he sought refuge in Switzerland, where he spent the rest of his life treating the needy. Sometimes he stroked their aching limbs to give them relief, and even sufferers from violent convulsions would pass into a deep sleep. He claimed that in his apartment, which he called 'la salles des crises', the evil in the body was released and, on waking, patients found that their symptoms had vanished. Some patients had merely to sit on a chair over which he passed his hands, to be either calmed or convulsed, and there is no doubt that he possessed phenomenal ability to convey suggestion which helped to cure disease. See: Hypnosis, Hypnotism.

Messegues, Maurice. Born 14.12.1921 at 4.30 p.m. at Calayrac-St Circq (Lot et Garonne), France, where he is the most renowned herbalist in the country. His father was also a herbalist, known as 'The Plant Expert,' who cured, among others, the local doctor Lapeyre from prostrate trouble. His father's knowledge influenced him for he was sent into the fields and woods to collect herbs and was taught how to make them into tisanes, poultices and other remedies. The famous as well as the poor and unknown beat a path to his door. Many were well

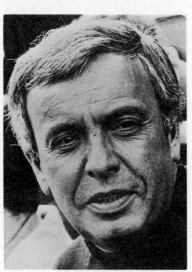

Maurice Messegues

known artistes: Nina Raya, Maurice Chevalier, Rina Ketty, Pierre Des, Charles Trenet and Mistinguett, to name a few. The highest in the land visited him: Admiral Darlan and President Herriot. He even advised Churchill and prescribed for him between 1950-57 but as soon as the old man was relieved of his ailments he went back to his wicked ways.

In France, as in America, herbalists are looked at askance by the medical profession and in 1945 he was prosecuted. He was prosecuted again and again till eventually a succession of medical men who were his clients gave evidence in his favour. At his last prosecution, though found guilty, his fine was halved. Then, because public opinion was strongly in his favour and men with household names such as Utrillo, Robert Schumann, Rockefeller, Adenauer, Cocteau and Prince Aly Khan sought relief in herbs when orthodox medicine had failed, the Medical Council ceased to persecute him. His methods differ from those of most herbalists for he cured not only by tisanes and infusions but by herbal foot and hip baths and compresses, and his book *Of Men and Plants* gives detailed instruction for making up his prescriptions. See: Herbalism.

Middle Eye See: Pineal gland.

Miles, Eustace. Former classical scholar of King's College, Cambridge; Assistant Master at Rugby School; coach and lecturer at Cambridge University. English tennis champion in 1899 and Champion of America at raquets and tennis in 1900, and Champion of England at raquets in 1902. A pioneer of *vegetarianism* and balanced diet. He started the famous Eustace Miles Restaurant in Chandos Street, Charing Cross, which provided excellent meatless meals, and founded one of the first physical culture schools in London. His wife ran the Eustace Miles School of Cookery, and both gave advice about diet, breathing, exercises and mental health at the Old House, Hemel Hempstead; and by correspondence. Miles devised a system of physical culture and he and his wife poured out a stream of pamphlets and books on vegetarianism, various aspects of health, and even reincarnation.

He invented Emprote, a food that has stood the test of time, and recently Appleford's who run a health food factory at Colnbrook, commemorated Eustace Miles by installing an action bronze of him playing tennis. He was one of the most gifted apostles of vegetarianism.

Milk. From time immemorial the cow, goat, ass, mare and camel have provided milk for human consumption and though it is not Man's natural food, it has served him well and he can live in perfect health on a lacto-vegetarian diet. It is a poor substitute for mother's milk in the feeding of infants, however, as its quality varies. In spring it is much richer in fat than in winter; and it must be diluted and sugar added, to make it quantitatively like mother's milk. Even then cow's milk is not the same because the principal protein, known as caseinogen, forms heavy curd, whereas the protein in human milk curdles into small, easily digested flocculi. Human milk also contains far more citric acid and less calcium, which also makes it more digestible than cow's milk. Moreover, the lactalbumin in cow's milk often causes eczema in small children. For infants there is no adequate substitute for human milk and none of the proprietary foods can compare with it.

Milk is not a 'perfect food' for there is no such thing. It stands high on the list of essential foods, however, as it contains all the amino-acids needed for life and growth. Its fats are easily digested by most people and it contains *riboflavin, vitamin A, K, and a little B₁, C and D*. It is rich in potassium, phosphorus, chlorine and calcium, but poor in iron. Cow's milk contains 87.30% water, 3.55% protein, 8.95% fat, 6.25% carbohydrates and 0.45% mineral salts. If only milk were taken, too much would be needed each day so, though not a perfect food, it is an excellent supplement. Two pints a day are recommended for growing children as milk influences weight and height, strengthens bone structure and protects the teeth from caries. As it is deficient in carbohydrates milk should be eaten with oats, whole grain bread, cereals and other carbohydrate foods. For convalescents it has few equals as it is swallowed easily, quenches thirst and is body-building; but it is a food and not a drink and invalids should sip it slowly and at intervals and eat it with a ripe banana. It should not be taken by adults as a drink for it is not easily absorbed –less so than any animal food. The large amount of water it contains interferes with absorption if taken as the sole food. It is much more easily absorbed by children than by adults, and with most difficulty by the aged.

It has been discovered during the last few years that some cannot digest milk easily because they have a deficiency of the digestive *enzyme* lactose (milk sugar) and children should never be forced to drink milk if they cannot keep it down. There are also an increasing number who are *allergic* to milk, perhaps because of the *hormones* with which cows are now injected, and break out in rashes, ulcers and itching of the skin. It has been found that 90% of the eczema in children is caused by an excessive consumption of milk products – except *yogurt;* and many adults with multiple sclerosis have improved when they gave up milk. Milk products and milk chocolate should not be given to sufferers from catarrh and bronchitis as no food forms mucous so rapidly. See: Yogurt, Cheese.

Milk, Dried. Dried skimmed milk contains all the elements present in full-cream milk except fat and vitamin B₁. It is far more easily assimilated than whole-milk and is a much better food for the elderly and for those who need to keep down their weight.

Milk Substitutes. Those who are allergic to milk products need not fear that their bodies will be deprived of calcium, phosphorus and potassium, so essential for the bones. Most of them can digest *yogurt.* For *vegans,* who object to animal products, there is plant milk. There is plenty of food rich in calcium, phosphorus and potassium: nuts, collards, kale, turnips, greens of every sort, egg yolk, *molasses, soya beans and soya flour, wholewheat* flour products, *seeds,* sardines, *agar-agar,* kelp and *lentils.*

Millet. A cereal consumed mainly in North Africa, being the staple food of tribes on the Upper Nile and in some southern European countries. In China it is used to make bread. Indian millet (sorgho-grass) is also a staple food in some parts of the country. Millet consists of 11.50% water, 9.00% protein, 3.80% fat, 70.20% carbohydrates, and 1.95% mineral matter.

Mineral Elements. Often referred to as 'mineral salts'. Although they comprise only about 5.00% of the body, without them the organs would not function. A man weighing 150 lb would have about 1050 grammes of calcium, 700 of phosphorus, 245 of potassium, 175 of sulphur, 105 of chlorine, 105 of sodium, 35 of magnesium, 2.8 of iron, 0.21 of manganese, 0.028 of iodine and traces of cobalt, silicon, silver, aluminium, arsenic, boron, copper, fluorine, nickel, zinc, lead, lithium, bromine, lanthanum, neodymium, cerium, tin, vanadium, chromium, rubidium, strontium, molybdenum, argon, beryllium, helium, neon, scandium and titanium.

The 'trace elements' exist in microscopic quantities: nickel, cobalt and lead in the pancreas; tin in the suprenal capsules; zinc in the liver and kidneys; silver in the uterus, ovaries, thyroid; heart, spleen and kidneys; aluminium in the lungs, kidneys, heart, testicles and pancreas; chromium in all the organs but mainly in the thyroid and spleen; copper in the lungs, liver and heart; tin an abundance in all organs; titanium mainly in the lungs; and zinc principally in the genital organs and thyroid. Analyses reveal that at least 40 of the 90 or more elements in sea-water are to be found in the body. The functions of the main minerals are known but those of most of the trace elements have yet to be discovered. We know, however, that the absence of some trace elements means all the difference between health and disease in plants and animals. If the soil is deficient in trace elements disease follows.

Mineral Waters. Mineral waters in Britain are of two types: (1) those to which chemical salts have been added, such as soda water, medical soda water, potash water, magnesia water, Carara water, Lithia water and Seltzer; (2) those which well from natural springs and can be sampled on the spot, as in Bath, Cheltenham, Leamington, Malvern etc., or are bottled and sold to the public.

Mind, Power of The. The most important factor in health is the mind for 90% of disease is psycho-somatic. This was realised centuries ago by physicians in India, China, Egypt, Ancient Greece and Rome, and by the Hebrews. The Arabs laid great stress on a patient's mental condition. Ideas originate in the mind and the thoughts they produce develop *emotions*, good and bad. Emotions have the effect of discharging *hormones* into the bloodstream. If harmful they poison the blood; if beneficial they produce healthy reactions.

Every action is preceded by thought followed by emotion and the results over the years are etched on the face, which is a reflection of the personality. The expression of a person is a true picture of his character and state of health, though many try to disguise this.

The ability to fight for health, or survival in extreme cases, is of paramount importance; and the patient's belief that he will recover is the doctor's greatest ally. Often a patient at death's door, who has been given up, refuses to die and because he has the will to live, recovers; sometimes only temporarily to see a project through, or a close relative who is late in arriving. Once the project is successful, or the relative has arrived, the patient relapses and dies.

Fear is the greatest opponent of health and does more to undermine resistance than anything. It conjures up the unknown, which is far more serious and frightening than reality. There are innumerable instances of fear alone causing death. A. W. T. Simeons, MD, says in *Man's Presumptuous Brain* that cholera, for instance, is caused by a microbe called a vibrio, known to be highly sensitive to acids, which are always present in the normal stomach. Fear and panic stops the flow of these acids and the alkaline condition allows the germ to breed. This is what often happens; people in areas where cholera is raging are overcome with fear and fall victims to the disease.

The sick should be placed in pleasant surroundings and their nurses should be not only efficient, but happy. If they are pretty as well, so much the better, for optimism is part of any cure. Henry de Mondeville (1260-1320) advised his pupils: 'Let the surgeon take care to regulate the regimen of the patient's life for joy and happiness by promising that he will soon be well, by allowing his relatives and special friends to cheer him and by having someone to tell him jokes [even if he eats his grapes!] and let him be solaced by music on the viol and psaltery. The surgeon should forbid anger, hatred and sadness in his patient, and remind him that the body grows fat from joy and thin from sadness. . . .'

In India the *kaviraj* (practitioner of Ayruvedic medicine) invariably greets his patient by asking: 'And how is your mind, temper and outlook today?' Happiness and contentment are the finest of all medicaments, and care and consideration the finest of salves.

Molasses. Thick black molasses with a slightly bitter flavour is, according to Dr S. C. Roy of the Indian Central Sugarcane Committee, 'both a food and a medicine'. It is mildly laxative, warms the body more than sugar, and can with advantage be given to mothers during lactation. In India it is prescribed by physicians of traditional medicine for *stomach* and *blood* ailments, bile disorders and *rheumatism*. It contains *aneurin, riboflavin, nicotinic acid, pantothenic acid, inositol* and *choline,* and is rich in the minerals *iron, calcium, magnesium, potassium, sodium, sulphur, chlorine* and *phosphorus.*

Molasses is the product of the first process of refining the juice of the sugar cane; further refinement produces Barbadoes sugar, Demerara sugar and finally *white sugar,* a dead product and an irritant.

Unlike refined sugar and treacle which tend to destroy the teeth, molasses according to Dr F. A. Stirling of New York, strengthens them. After studying the eating habits of West Indians and Africans he wrote: 'The coloured race, particularly those living on whole corn meal and a molasses diet of the southern plantations, have good teeth.'

Molasses can be taken in many ways: in warm water or milk; on porridge or wheat germ; with yogurt; spread on bread; or in cakes and puddings instead of sugar. It is not a cathartic but a dessertspoon of molasses added to a tablespoon or two of *bran* and warm milk each day will relieve stubborn cases of constipation.

Mono Diet. During the thirties some food reformers advocated the consumption of one kind of food only, at each meal; that is, either meat or bread or porridge or fruit or vegetables and nothing else. A few adhered to it for a while and maintained good health but it was far too monotonous to make many converts and restricted one's social life, and was soon forgotten.

Moxabustion. Part of the treatment in Chinese *acupuncture*. The practitioner prepares tiny balls of *moxa,* made from leaves of the Chinese wormwood tree, which are ignited and placed on the relevant points. They are allowed to burn down till they touch the skin, when they are removed by the practitioner, who crushes the ashes into the skin as he does so. Moxa is used either alternately or in conjunction with the needles.

Moxibustion. The Ancients found that sometimes accidental burns cured insanity and cauterised patients on the neck and head with branding irons, selecting spots according to precise rules. Albucasis, the famous Arab physician, wrote what is perhaps the first book on 'fire surgery' in which he said that piercing the lobe of the ear with a pointed branding iron often cured vertigo and defective hearing. The Geneva physician Gonin pricked the eyeball with a red-hot iron to cure detachment of the retina, and Arab doctors cured various diseases by burning spots on the temples, forehead, back of the neck and ears, and on the eyelids. Dr *Aschner* relates that a physician in an oriental city told him of an Arab youth who went to him with an inflamed and infected arm. 'See me tomorrow,' he told the lad but the boy failed to return. When he saw him in the street not long after, he asked why he had failed to turn up. 'I could not afford the operation,' confessed the boy, 'so I went to a lay healer, who drew a fine line with a red-hot iron round my wrist, and the swelling and pain vanished.' Possibly the cauterised line blocked off the lymph vessels and reduced pain and infection, without resort to surgery. Cauterisation is also practised by Ayurvedic physicians in India.

Muller, Lieut. J. P. Former lieutenant in the Danish Army who was a follower of *Rikli*. He believed that fresh air, sunlight and deep breathing were the foundations of health. His ideas were incorporated into a book entitled *My System* and he founded the Health and Strength League under the patronage of the Prince of Wales, which had more than 100,000 members in Britain alone. Muller maintained that the skin and lungs were the most important organs and that exercise, which strengthened the heart, should always be performed either in the open, or in a room with wide-open windows. He wrote a number of books on *sun bathing* and the value of breathing and fresh air which had a wide sale in Britain, the Continent, and throughout the Empire. He believed that exercise and exposure of the naked body to air and sunlight hardened it, and many who came to him with tuberculosis after the orthodox system had failed them, were restored to health.

Mushroom. Till recently mushrooms were valued only for the flavour they imparted to food, and all but the common mushroom *(Psalliota campestris)* and the Horse Mushroom were believed to be poisonous.

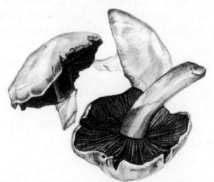

There are, however, about 30 varieties of mushroom which are edible: shaggy cap, the blusher, the parasol, the ragged parasol, blewits, St. George's mushroom, the oyster, fairy rings, champignon, chanterelle, saffron milk cap, the giant puff ball, boletus and the morel being the best known.

Mushrooms are rich in vitamin B and D and the French say they render one immune to cancer because French mushroom growers have been free from this disease for more than 100 years. Mushrooms have been eaten by the Hebrews since biblical times and by the Chinese, Japanese and Indians for centuries, and used by all four in drugs for curing certain diseases and fighting bacterial infection. This has been endorsed by Dr Alfred Hayes, bacteriologist at the Glasshouse Crops Research Institute, Littlehampton, who states that they contain *riboflavin, thiamin, niacin* and *folic acid*. Dr Arthur Karler believes they contain a good quality protein and if grown in sufficient quantity could feed millions of under-nourished people. The truffle, a type of fungus like the mushroom, sells for more than £80 a lb.

Music, The Therapeutic Value of. Though music has played a part in curing disease – especially disease of the mind – since the earliest times it has only recently been recognised for its remedial qualities in Europe and America. The Israelites played music in their temples and the Bible tells us that 'David took a harp and played music with his hand; so Saul was refreshed and well, and the evil spirit departed from him'. In Ancient India immense importance was placed on *mantras* and temple music and their priests said: 'Sounds made by humans can carry an influence of mind over matter.' In Ancient Greece Apollo, God of Music, was also God of Medicine. Hippocrates took patients to the temple to listen to music and Aristotle spoke and wrote about its healing effects on mind and body. The Ancient Egyptians, whose medicine is based on that of the Assyrians and Babylonians, used music to cure as long ago as 1600 BC and their melodies were played to sufferers from sciatica, *rheumatism* and other pains which drugs failed to alleviate; and for insect bites.

Thomas Cogan and Richard Browne, physicians famous in the sixteenth and seventeenth centuries used music in their practices; and Berlioz, Borodin and Boyd Neel, who started life as doctors, believed in the curative power of music – as did Albert Schweitzer.

The first modern to incorporate music into his philosophy was *Steiner*, the founder of Anthroposophy. Today it is generally accepted by the medical profession that music has a significant part to play in curing a variety of diseases and it is widely used in mental hospitals, and for handicapped children. The normal person, in sickness and health, can also gain infinite refreshment from music, which in some instances has a hypnotic effect and in others may act as an anaesthetic, and operations have been performed under the influence of music.

Music can have either a stimulating or tranquillising effect, depending on the kind played; and some kinds of music can temporarily add new life and vigour. The greatest value, however, lies in its soothing effect which dissipates stress, banishes worry and pain and does much to counteract the pressures of modern life.

Mustard Oil. Mustard is a valuable crop, bearing a seed which when crushed provides flour. When mixed with water this forms a paste much used as a condiment; when strongly diluted and added to a foot-bath helps to ward off colds and chills. Mustard oil forms the basis of many unguents and embrocations, and Pliny wrote: 'It is so pungent in taste that it burns like fire although at the same time it is remarkably wholesome for the body.' Pythagoras used it as an antidote to scorpion bites and in Old England a potent cough cure was concocted by boiling powdered mustard with figs in strong ale. In India it has been used for centuries as an ingredient in curries and, mainly in Bengal curries are cooked in mustard oil.

According to *Diet and Food Reform* by M. K. Gandhi, the oil contains 99% of fat together with traces of manganese, nickel and cobalt; and if the human skin, which contains ergosterol, is rubbed with it and exposed to the sun, it is rapidly converted into vitamin D. Without knowing this Bengali mothers have from time immemorial rubbed their infants all over with mustard oil and put them out in the morning sun.

N

Nails. The appearance of the nails indicates the general state of health and in the past family doctors always examined a patient's nails. Today with so many instant drugs available such an insignificant item is usually overlooked.

Nails, like every other part of the body, receive their nourishment from the blood and if the diet is faulty the result will often be apparent in the condition of the nails. One of the most common symptoms is the fluted nail, which means that the system is out of balance, for the surface of the nail from tip to base should be smooth, and either fluting or ridging is a sign of nervous disorder. So is brittleness, which means that the blood lacks silica.

White spots or flecks are warnings to people with delicate nerves and indicate stress and a loss of vitality. Very short nails indicate a quick temper and a critical nature, often brought about by bad health.

If the nails tend to turn back it indicates a degree of nervous destruction or mental disorder, and if they are fluted as well nervous prostration is likely. A nail with a distinct horizontal ridge indicates damage and a sign that one nail has died and another is replacing it. This usually happens when a nail has received a sharp blow or been caught in the jamb of a door and becomes bloodshot. As it takes about six months for a nail to grow from base to tip the date of the accident can be calculated.

A ridge across the nail also indicates a serious illness or accident to the body, and again you can judge how long ago the illness took place.

Nails that are scooped out like saucers with the tips tending to turn back indicate serious nervous conditions, and unless steps are taken to rectify diet and the way of life, nervous prostration is likely, and in extreme cases, paralysis.

The bulbous nail on a bulbous finger tip is usually a sign of pulmonary trouble such as tuberculosis. The nail also has a bluish tinge indicating bad circulation or congestion of blood. This does not mean that TB is present but a severe cold or chill may set events in motion that will cause it.

Nails may be blue, red, yellowish or purple. Each colour denotes some malfunctioning of the body and these in conjunction with ridges, flecks, spots, etc., point either to ill health or impending illness. Healthy nails should be smooth, pink and without blemishes. One must, of course, make allowances for age as after middle age nails tend to become increasingly thick and tough, and often, brittle, especially where the person has arteriosclerosis or varicose veins, or both. Diabetics should take care to have their nails pared regularly as gangrene can result from in-growing toe nails which pierce the skin.

Nature Cure. Ambroise Pare the famous French surgeon, who was the first to abandon the practice of pouring boiling oil into gunshot wounds, said: 'I dressed him and God healed him.' and Sir *William Osler,* the leading English-speaking physician of his day, said that Nature alone healed and the best that any doctor could do was to help Nature.

Nature Cure is based on the principle that the body is a self-healing organism and, if during illness it is rested, fasted, and then given the right sort of food in small quantities, increasing as health improves, all diseases can be cured, till eventually the body wears out with old age. Osler said that 'One of the most striking characteristics of modern treatment of disease is the return to what used to be called natural methods –*diet, exercise, bathing* and *massage.* There probably never was a period in the history of the profession when the value of diet in the prevention and the cure of disease has been more fully recognised.

Dr. Joseph Kidd wrote in *Laws of Therapeutics*: 'Medicine is yet to a great extent a mere collection of facts and opinions which vary from year to year, according to the theories of the most prominent men.'

From time to time medical men have come to the fore with theories for perfect health, the prolongation of life and the cure of disease, but none of these theories existed for any length of time. According to *J. H. Kellogg*, Professor Atwater, the leading American authority on 'scientific diet' and an advocate of high-protein diet, died of atereosclerosis at a comparatively early age after living for nearly three years as a completely helpless, imbecile paralytic.

One could fill a book with quotations by eminent medical men who have criticised modern medical methods, the propensity to prescribe *drugs* for almost every ailment, and operations where more often than not none were necessary. Medicine has taken the wrong turning and become more 'scientific' instead of working with Nature. Every disease can be cured if taken in hand in time and the conditions that cause it are removed. Causes and not symptoms, are what matter, and Nature sets out to eradicate the causes.

In Nature Cure the first step is nearly always a fast while the body is rested; when the blood is cleared of impurities the patient has a chance to recover. To aid the healing process the Naturopath will give water or water with fruit juices, followed by a diet of fresh fruit, salads, conservatively cooked vegetables and *proteins* in the form of eggs, cheese and nuts. Vitamins from natural sources may be prescribed, together with hot and cold compresses and baths. *Herbs* may be administered as tisanes and infusions, and *homeopathy, acupuncture, osteopathy* and *chiropractic* may all be used as aids to further the healing process. The naturopath will decide which treatment will best help *fasting* and *diet*. *Hypnosis* may also be used.

The body always returns to health if it is treated as a whole' and not in separate parts independent of the rest. This is the principle on which Nature Cure rests and because it is fundamentally sound gains more adherents from the ranks of thinking people every year.

Naturopath. Practitioner of Natural methods of healing.

Naturopathy. The science and art of curing by natural methods.

Nettle *(Urtica Dioca)*. The sight of the common stinging nettle enrages most gardeners, who dig out and burn it not realising its value as a vegetable, a medicinal aid, and as a means of adding heat to the compost heap. The nettle is rich in *iron, sulphur, calcium, sodium* and *vitamin C*. In spring the tops of young nettles (about four inches) boiled, taste very much like spinach and are much superior as a food. The water, drained off, can be used as stock. Nettles and seawrack boiled together, are good for slimming. If the boiled leaves are made into a compress and applied externally they will stop bleeding almost instantly, and a nettle poultice if not left on too long, will relieve pain. The water from boiled nettles will expel worms and a tea made from the roots is good for the lungs, intestines, stomach and nose, and will stop haemorrage of the urinary organs.

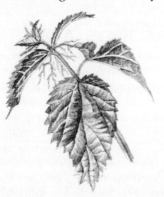

Few herbs equal the nettle as a hair tonic, which restores the colour of the hair and cures dandruff. The leaves should be boiled in either water or vinegar and the liquid rubbed into the scalp daily. There is no part of the nettle which cannot be used: the seeds and flowers macerated in wine were once a specific for ague; an infusion of nettle, wild cherry and blackberry root are good for bowel troubles; and the juice of nettles is good for constipation, rheumatism and gout.

The fine hairs on the nettle contain formic acid and when touched inject this into the skin, causing a stinging sensation. John Parkinson, the King's Herbalist in 1640 said that Roman soldiers in Britain used nettles 'to rubbe and chafe their limbs when through extreme cold they should be stiffe and benumbed'. The writer has never tried that but he has had his back stroked by nettles to cure lumbago and a leg stroked to relieve sciatica; in both instances the cure was instantaneous and no stinging was felt! Flogging the back with nettles is a recognised treatment for rheumatic troubles and lumbago in Poland and parts of Eastern Europe. Pepys wrote in February 1661: 'We did eat some nettle porridge... which was very good'. Nettle brews and nettle beer are tasty and good for the health. They cleanse the blood and recipes for making them appeared in many Victorian cookery books. A bunch of nettles hung in a larder will soon drive out all flies.

There are some 500 varieties of nettles. Those in Europe are harmless and have medicinal properties but in South-East Asia there are kinds, which if touched will cause a sting that lasts for a year and may even result in death. The British nettle is a much under-valued herb: in 1917 the Germans made socks, great-coats and tarpaulins for trucks out of nettles, and in the 1939 war the Nazis imported 5,000 trucks of them for their textile indus-try.

Noise. Vibrations conveyed through the atmosphere which impinge on the hearing apparatus of the ear. If this is destroyed as in the case of the totally deaf, noise ceases to exist. The audible range of sound varies from 16 to 20,000 cycles and though the correct unit of measurement is the *phon,* the decibel is the commonly accepted measure. The threshold of hearing is zero and leaves gently rustling in the wind, ten. The danger level of noise starts at 80 decibels, which is the sound one has to endure inside a noisy car, a noisy office or in heavy traffic. The threshold of pain is 120, which is a billion times greater than the least audible sound. This is endured by workers in a boiler factory or those within 500 feet of a jet plane. Sound frequencies of 150 decibels can burn the skin, and 180 is a lethal level.

Sound is one of the most destructive elements of the present age, though fortunately the human ear has a remarkable ability to accustom itself to sound in volume and the middle ear pre-vents the transmission of waves of excessive intensity to the inner ear, and so saves the ear drum from rupture. Continuous loud noise over prolonged periods, however, as in a discothe-que, thickens the bones of the inner ear and causes deafness, whereas a little excessive noise can, on occasion, stimulate. Long exposure to noise will destroy health by causing tinnitus, dizziness, headaches, nausea, and fullness in the ears, and in the case of sensitive persons fear of excessive noise can have the same effect.

Tests show that women though not impervious to noise endure it with greater equanimity than men and in many fac-tories where the noise level is comparatively high, grow accus-tomed to it. It has been proved that noise in places of work reduces efficiency, and where intricate work is done, results in more errors being made than is normal. In a survey carried out by the Alfred Marks Bureau in 1974 in which 1,000 employees took part, it was found that 46% complained of headaches, 38% of backaches, 33% of eye strain, and 15% of aching wrists. In badly planned offices 23% developed neuroses and 42% suffered from impaired efficiency.

Homes, factories, offices and even roads are plagued with noise which grows in intensity each year. The medical authorities in all large cities are alarmed at the effect it has on general health and efficiency and fear that unless world-wide drastic action is taken *psychomatic* diseases will increase on a vast scale, or people will grow deaf, for deafness is Nature's defence against noise.

Noise acts like a drug. There is no condition to which the body adjusts itself so easily, and therein lies its deadliness. Increasing noise can be accepted with equanimity till a limit is reached when the body can stand it no longer and breaks down. Till recently noise has not been associated with stress and fatigue, but now we know that it can cause actual physical sickness. It is such a destructive force that unless means can be found to silence cars, planes and noisy machines, the survival of the human race is threatened.

Nose. The nose is an organ of smell, the most subtle of our senses, and the mechanism of the nose is able to receive an unlimited number of odour stimulii. The greatest value of smell is to perceive stenches which warn us of rotting matter which is unfit to be eaten, and so saves us from food poisoning. The nose also warns of danger for it senses smoke, burning wood, paint and other combustibles; it gives warning of poisonous fumes such as those given off by petrol, paraffin and other liquids.

The nose tells us of the presence of many things long before we can see them: new mown hay, burning peat, cigar smoke, roasting coffee, curry, fried onions, bacon, mushrooms, polished leather, certain kinds of wood, fish in bulk at a distance or fish being fried, manure, the presence of a sewage farm, and the proximity of the sea – sometimes even though it may be miles away. And of course, the scent of flowers and the perfumes which women use.

The nose is needed for the full enjoyment of food and it sets in motion gastric juices which aid digestion. If you block your nostrils and eat fish and chips or steak and onions much of the flavour of these dishes will be lost. In my youth we used to nip our nostrils with finger and thumb while castor oil was poured down our throats. The law recognises that a sense of smell is important to the enjoyment of life and on more than one occasion damages have been paid to people who have been deprived of it in road accidents.

The nose often indicates the first sign of ill health by losing its sense of smell or by becoming blocked, as happens in the case of an approaching cold or influenza. It is necessary, therefore, to keep it in good condition by proper breathing and a balanced *diet*.

Do not blow your nose through both nostrils at the same time as this tends to send matter which should be blown out, into the sinuses in your forehead. Block one nostril and blow through the other. If you wish to flush your nose by drawing water into it, close one nostril and draw the water into the other, then reverse the process. Then the water will pass through one nostril, into the connecting passage, and out through the other. See: Smell, Senses.

Nudism. Pioneers of the Naked Cult were Diefenbach, Guttzeit, Gust and Nagel, who was the most famous of all. He believed that Man was intended to go naked and set his face against the argument that Man was originally a tropical animal who through force of circumstances had wandered into temperate and frigid zones, so must wear clothes to protect his body from the cold. Nagel cited the case of the climate-hardened women of the Tierra del Fuego (one of the coldest habitable regions on earth) who wear nothing but a loin cloth and swim in the icebound sea; naked Eskimos in the Arctic Circle who entertained Frithjof Nansen in unheated mud huts. Several fanatics on the Continent adopted Nagel's ideas and, where the law allowed, went entirely naked, a condition which they claimed improved both their health and morality.

The Doubokors of Russia also went naked and when thousands of them emigrated to Canada they continued to practise nudism. Major Hans Suren, a German, was the foremost advocate of nudism after the First World War but his regimen was much too spartan for most people. The present Nudist Movement sprang from Suren, whose disciples wore their hair long, rejected shoes and socks and, when they went into public places covered their bodies with a long toga or cassock, tied at the neck, with holes for the arms.

Muller condemned complete nudity, however, and said that at least bathing slips should be worn. He argued that many who practised nudism had repulsive bodies, with too much fat and a course of physical culture was necessary before they exhibited their bodies.

Today nudism is practised on the shores of the Black Sea, in parts of Germany, France, Britain and America and the apostles of nudism are the better for it.

O

Oats. Oats are an excellent body building food, the whole oat more so than when ground into meal or rolled, when some of the fat may be lost. Oats contain more fat in an easily digested form than any other cereal, which makes them ideal for northern climates. They flourish mainly in temperate zones but have also been grown as far north as the Arctic Circle. For centuries they have been the staple food of the Scots. In Britain and America rolled oats are eaten mainly as a breakfast food together with milk or cream, and sugar; in Scotland coarse or whole oats were cooked in water and eaten with a sprinkle of salt. They also form the basis of haggis and a variety of cakes and biscuits peculiar to that country. Today oats form a part of all muesli products.

Oats can be taken in many forms. Oatmeal tea, made by boiling two tablespoons of coarse oatmeal in a quart of water for an hour and then adding the juice of two lemons and the grated rind of one, is a refreshing drink and in the past was provided by farmers for their workers at harvest time. Oatmeal jelly is good for children and invalids; and oatmeal porridge with a spoon of raw oatmeal sprinkled over it is a good laxative. Oat straw boiled for an hour and taken with a little honey, eases chest complaints. Homeopaths sometimes prescribe a tincture made from Black Oats for neuresthenia, general debility, fatigue and colds. Whole or coarse oats contain 12.40% water, 10.40% protein, 5.20% fat, 57.80% carbohydrates and 3.02% mineral matter, mainly *potassium* and *phosphorus*, together with *vitamins* B_1, B_2, *niacin*, *E*; and they are a good source of *iodine*.

Oats, Quaker. In the middle of the last century Americans devoured enormous breakfasts consisting of salt fish, beefsteak, sausages, boiled fowl, ham and bacon, corn bread in gravy, jam, honey, potatoes and other vegetables. European immigrants were staggered at the quantities they ate. In 1854 Ferdinand Schumacher, who arrived from Germany, decided to do something about this time consuming meal and ground oats into meal in a backroom of his grocery store at Akron, Ohio. Other Germans who had eaten oats at home, sent for his oatmeal, which he sold at first in bulk, then in jars. Every day he milled about 3,600 lb of oats and soon his German Mills American Oatmeal factory was thriving. In 1873 he published a cookery book containing recipes for oatmeal and in 1877 he issued an oatmeal breakfast cereal in a packet with the picture of a Quaker on it. By 1886 Schumacher owned the largest milling complex in the world and created a new industry with oatmeal as a substitute for protein. Then his mill was destroyed by fire and he was not insured! Later Robert Stuart started a similar mill 16 miles from Akron, also with the picture of a Quaker on the packet, and today the Quaker Oats Company has tentacles all over the world and sells half a billion dollars of cereal products – 200 varieties in all – of which Quaker Oats form the main food.

Oldfield, Dr Josiah (1863-1953). born in Andover, the son of a blind organist. Educated at Newport Grammar School. His ambition to enter Oxford was thwarted because his father could not afford the fees, so he worked as a junior master at his old school and by making every sacrifice saved £40; but as the fees were £300 a year he could gain admission only as an unattached scholar. He rented a room for ten shillings a week and lived on wholewheat bread and porridge, both sustaining foods, and in order to keep fit and make some money he took a job as stone-breaker and road-maker with the City Council at 6d an hour, working from 5.30 to 7.30 each morning. He had to

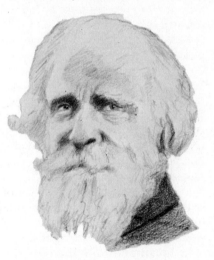

Dr Josiah Oldfield

obtain special permission to do so as no student is allowed to leave his rooms before six. Eventually Dr Kitchen came to his rescue and appointed him Visiting Mathematical Master to New

Olive

College Chorister School. In spite of severe handicaps he obtained a creditable degree in the Honours School in theology and law. After graduating he entered one of the Inns of Court, was called to the Bar and practised on the Oxford Circuit. His thesis on Capital Punishment earned him a doctorate of Civil Law and he founded the Society for the Abolition of Capital Punishment.

Oldfield was one of the first *fruitarians* in Britain and a *food reformer*. He did more than anyone to make people aware of the value of *honey* as a food, and he was a friend and associate of Shaw, Henry Salt, Allinson and others prominent in the food reform world. He worked vigorously almost to the age of 90.

Olive. The olive is a native of Asia, from where it spread to the Mediterranean and is now cultivated in North Africa, Australia, California and parts of South America. When ripe the fruit is black, and the finest quality olives grow on the Mediterranean coasts and North Africa, where 40-60% of the fruit is oil as compared with 25% in California. Spain and Italy are the two main olive growing countries. When ripe the fruit is bitter. Green olives are used exclusively for pickling. Ripe olives are dried and eaten in a variety of ways, and for export they are pickled in brine. They contain the maximum quantity of oil just before they are ripe and the highest quality of olive oil comes from hand-picked fruit which is dried and then pressed gently. The oil is golden or straw-coloured and has neither smell nor taste. Subsequent pressings have a greenish tint. Olive oil should always be kept in opaque containers for when it is exposed to sunlight it becomes rancid and develops an offensive odour. The olive is a good food containing oil in a highly digestible form, and it is best eaten with salads or in combination with other fruit. The oil is both a food and a medicine and one of the best sources of fat as it is said to reduce cholesterol in the arteries.

In Spain and Italy the oil is heated and bread with garlic rubbed in it, is dropped into the oil, simmered for a few seconds, then drained and eaten, usually with tomatoes or strips of cucumber. The oil is a gentle aperient and a tablespoonful may be given to young children with salads.

The oil is good for sufferers from debility or those who are

116

under-weight, and if their digestions rebel at taking it in its pure form, it should be put into half a pint of milk, water added, and whisked. Honey added, makes it palatable.

There is no oil, except perhaps mustard oil, as good for the skin for it is easily absorbed into the subcutaneous layers, keeps the skin supple and the body flexible and pliant. Unfortunately the first pressings of olive oil are difficult to get in Britain. The dried olive contains 30.07% water, 5.24% protein, 51.90% fat, 10.45% carbohydrates, and 2.33% mineral matter, being exceptionally rich in potassium.

Onion. The onion is a favourite herb in British cookery and steak-and-onions and tripe-and-onions are traditional dishes. The raw onion has little smell but when eaten raw, taints the breath. When cooked, however, it leaves no offensive odour and the smell of onions being fried is one of the most appetising known to man. It sets the gastric juices working.

Onions are among the oldest herbs known and were eaten in large quantities by the Israelites when they were building the pyramids: 'We remember the fish which we did eat in Egypt freely; the cucumbers and the melons, and the leeks and the onions and the garlick.' (Numbers 40.5). Onions grew wild in Egypt and were eaten in the desert as a preventive against thirst.

Priests and holy men discovered the medicinal properties of the onion and incorporated it into plasters for aches and pains and rheumatism, beat it into suet and administered it for wasting diseases, poured the juice into aching ears, and prescribed it for skin complaints. Docorides, Galen and Pliny the Elder, and the Arab physicians el Israilly and Rhazes valued it for its healing properties. The Ancient Hindus set much store on the onion, and so did the herbalists Culpepper and Gerarde. In 1910 Dr Mangor, and in 1912 Dr Dalche, and during the 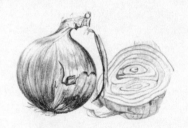 First World War Dr Leclerc, published papers on onions and their effects on specific diseases and found after conducting scores of experiments, that the essential oils of the onion and *garlic* (and certain strongly scented herbs), kill bacteria. They called the elusive element *phytonicides*. The antiseptic properties lie in the smell for when the onion is peeled and cut and the odour evaporates, so does the phytonicides. Scientists at the University of California also claim to have isolated this element, which they call *allyl aldehyde*. About 50 years ago Luther Burbank the famous plant breeder, produced an odourless onion, but it lacked flavour, housewives said it tasted like a tulip bulb and refused to buy it. It also lacked *phytonicides*.

Soviet scientists ground onions and garlic into pulp, put them into open tubes and applied the ends to wounds and septic sores that refused to heal. Though none of the pulp was in contact with the wounds this vapourised treatment healed them after two or three applications of from two to ten minutes.

The onion also possesses antiscorbutic properties, is good for the skin and experiments at the Royal Victoria Infirmary, Newcastle, suggest that onions can prevent blood clotting and are an antidote to some heart conditions; and it is well known that people who eat raw onions regularly are singularly free from colds and chills. An onion a day, preferably raw, will do much to keep the doctor away. The onion consists of 87.60% water, 1.60% protein, 0.30% fat, 9.90% carbohydrates, and 0.60% mineral matter, mainly potassium, calcium, phosphorus and silicon.

Orange. The orange is native of the Middle East and was introduced into England during the Crusades. It was cultivated in Spain by the Moors who over-ran North Africa, Spain and France up to Avignon, and seeds were taken to the West Indies and the Americas by the colonists.

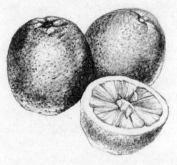

It was valued in Britain for its fragrance and health-giving properties for in his *Haven of Health* (1584), Thomas Cogan the famous physician and herbalist wrote: 'The rinds of oranges are preserved condite in sugar, and so are the flowers of the orange tree. Either of them being taken in a little quantity do greatly comfort a feeble stomach', and to this day orange peel retains its place as a stomachic cordial in the pharmacopæia.

In Pepys' day oranges were a luxury, costing 6d each (a considerable sum) and in Tudor times they were cultivated by landed gentry in specially built orangeries and the fruit served

118

either raw or boiled, with meats; they were used also for flavouring fish and eggs. Their value as an antiscorbutic was not realised till *James Lind* wrote his famous treatise. The orange is an alkaliniser and the juice given to young children ensures that the dentine on teeth is deposited evenly, so that they have smooth surfaces on which deposits of food will not lodge. The orange must be picked when ripe for it will never ripen, no matter how long it is kept, if picked when green or yellow-green. Green specks on a ripe orange, however, mean that when it ripened the weather was unusually hot. The orange contains 86.90% water, 0.80% protein, 0.20% fat (most of the oil is in the skin), 11.60% carbohydrates, and 0.50% mineral salts, mainly potassium and calcium.

Osler, Sir William. (1849-1919). The most celebrated English-speaking physician of his day and an inspiring teacher. Born in Canada of English parents, graduated at McGill University and studied at Glasgow, Vienna, Edinburgh and Berlin, was Professor of Medicine successively at Montreal, Philadelphia, Baltimore and Oxford. His magnificent library of valuable medical works was bequeathed to McGill. He wrote a number of books, articles and papers, and his best known *Principle and Practice of Medicine* is still not outdated.

Osler believed that only Nature can cure and the most that doctors can do is to assist.

Oslo Meal. At various times composite meals containing all the necessary nutriments have been put forward as 'perfect'. One such was the Oslo Meal devised during World War II, when many essential foods were scarce. It was given to school children and consisted of 100% wholewheat bread, butter, cheese, salad and fruit and it was claimed that the meal would render them resistant to disease and prevent dental caries. The Oslo Meal, so named after the city where it was first tried out, contains the vitamins B-complex, A, C and D which are provided by fresh salads and grated carrot, herbs in season, fresh fruit and oranges. Yeast extract was sprinkled over the salad and eggs were included when available (the ration was one a month!).

An experiment was tried with 100 children, 50 of whom were given an Oslo Meal every day while the other 50 were fed on the usual cooked food common in their homes. At the end of the trial period those on the Oslo Meal increased by more than 25% in height and weight over those not on the diet. Moreover, the children on the Oslo Meal suffered far fewer of the normal ailments common to the young. The Oslo Meal was not always the same. Variations were devised with, for instance, a boiled egg, two substantial slices of wholewheat bread and an ounce (!) of butter, a tomato, a glass of milk and a banana, which provided a balanced meal.

Osteopathy. A method of manipulation devised by *Dr Andrew Still* who founded the College of Osteopathy at Kirksville, Missouri, in 1892. 'To find health', said Still, 'should be the object of the osteopath. Anyone can find disease.'

He said that the structure determines function; that is, if parts of the body are out of alignment they will not function efficiently and it is the task of the osteopath to rectify this. Disease is usually due to the wrong sort of diet, which affects various parts of the body and it is the task of the osteopath to manipulate the spine if it is out of alignment, break down lesions and return the body to its normal state. But if the diet is again neglected the same troubles will return.

Sometimes joints lock round a sprain and the ligaments round the joint are in tension and intense agony is caused if they are stretched. The nerve ends send out impulses to the brain, giving a sensation of pain; the blood supply is affected altering the size of the blood vessels and the nerve supply to the area around the joint and to those reflexly connected to them.

The osteopath firmly but gently unlocks the joint and moves it back to its normal position by using techniques he has been taught. This reduces pain, causes a normal flow of blood, releases nerves or nerve ends that may be pinched and restores the body to a healthy state. The muscles, ligaments, connective tissue etc., must be encouraged – not forced – back to normal, and treatment in every case is governed by the nature of the patient. Treatment can be given to babies under six months and to the very aged, depending on the nature of the tissues, nervous disposition and constitutional make-up.

In the public mind the osteopath is associated with the cure of stiff necks, slipped discs, low back pains, cartilages and joints out of place, sprained ankles, sciatica, tennis elbow and frozen shoulders, etc. The orthodox practitioners put patients into plastic collars and rigid waistcoats, immobilising the affected parts in the hope that time will heal, whereas the osteopath, using special techniques, sometimes cures within minutes.

What is not generally known is that the osteopath and the *chiropractor* can cure tonsilitis, alleviate heart attacks, stomach troubles, rheumatism and arthritis, and many nervous diseases by manipulations which increase the supply of blood and release irritated nerves. Dr McDonald and Dr Hargrave-Wilson, two of Still's early disciples, proved that misalignment of the spinal bones and joints, ligaments and muscles, affect internal organs. When they are brought into line health can usually be restored if the disease has not progressed too far. But in almost every case it can alleviate. Unfortunately, osteopaths and *chiropractors* often have to deal with patients who have been the round of doctors and failed to obtain relief.

Osteopathy is not recognised by the medical profession though many doctors go to osteopaths for treatment and it cannot be had on the NHS. Fifty years ago there were five flourishing osteopathic colleges in America: Kirksville, Chicago, Los Angeles, Des Moines and Philadelphia, where anatomy, physiology, chemistry, pathology, bacteriology, physiotherapy, surgery, the practice of medicine and diagnosis were taught. The average number of school hours was 4,953 whereas in the leading medical colleges the number was 4,542. Ninety years ago there was one osteopath in America; 70 years ago 18; 50 years ago 10,000. In 1902 they invaded Britain. In 1911 the British Osteopathic Association was formed and a register kept. By 1935 more than half a million people in Britain had been treated successfully and an attempt was made in Parliament to pass a Bill recognising osteopathy. But despite the backing of many prominent medical men – some in the House of Commons – the Act never became law. The resistance by the medical profession was too strong. Today osteopaths flourish as never before. In America the osteopath is known as an osteopathic physician, has a status equal to that of the MD and can diagnose, prescribe drugs, perform surgery and practice psychiatry.

P

P-Vitamin. See: Vitamin P.

Pain. Pain is a blessing in disguise for without it we would not know what has gone wrong with the body. In the case of a broken limb pain is felt at the site of the fracture, which can be seen; but internal pains cannot. Rheumatism and other twinges are alarm calls for action to be taken. Sometimes when a muscle is 'fixed' it shuts off its own blood supply and causes 'referred pain' at some distance from the muscle. Minor twinges are often ignored and are set right by the body's self-adjusting mechanism. Pain of any intensity, however, especially if it is frequent, calls for attention, and if ignored the consequences can be serious. Even an aching tooth should not be constantly alleviated by pain-killers and an appointment with the dentist should be made as soon as possible.

Painful impressions are conducted from the skin and organs by nerve fibres which, when they reach the spinal cord cross over and run upwards, ending in a large basal nucleus of the brain known as the thalmus. From here the impressions are relayed and sometimes amplified, to the cortical centres. There are a few unfortunate people who seem immune to pain, and another small group with a chronic disease called *Syringomyelia*; both groups can suffer serious illness without showing any symptoms and as a result are difficult to cure when assailed by disease. Their nerves do not respond as they do in normal people.

When undergoing a medical test your doctor will ask you to cross one leg over another and tap the overlapping knee with a mallet. If the leg jumps he knows that your nerves are in good order. Another test is to run a pointed instrument along the sole of your foot. Unless the foot is withdrawn quickly there is something wrong with the nerves. Pain cannot be measured in chemical terms. It is something we feel and react to spontaneously.

If you suffer from rheumatic pains, stomach ulcers, etc., consult your local naturopath, who is usually also an osteopath or a chiropractor. He will get to the seat of the trouble and relieve, and then cure it.

Palmer, Daniel David. Born of English-German parents in Port Perry, near Toronto. Emigrated to the US where he became interested in healing the sick and practised some of the many procedures then in vogue, among them *diet* and treatment by herbs. His investigations occupied many fields, among them manipulation of the body to restore circulation. He also practised 'magnetic healing' based on the discovery of animal magnetism, discovered by *Mesmer*, with great success. On 18th September 1896 a janitor named Harvey Lillard, who was so deaf that he could not hear the rumbling of waggons in the street, entered his office and asked for help. He explained that 17 years earlier while in a cramped stooping position he had suddenly exerted himself, felt something give way in his back, and lost his hearing. On examining him Palmer located a prominent vertebra which appeared out of place and reasoned that if it were put back the man's hearing might be restored. Using the spinous process of the vertebra as a lever, Palmer applied a short thrust with the butt of his hand which put the bone into position and soon after Lillard's hearing was normal again. This success made Palmer experiment with 'hand treatments'. He studied anatomy and by trial and error discovered the exact places in which to apply thrusts based on bone nerves and the manifestation of impulses. He was successful in relieving and curing a wide variety of ailments which did not respond to orthodox medical treatment and people travelled from far and wide to his surgery. With practise he improved his techniques and became the first healer to replace vertebrae by using the bony projections, the spinous and transverse processes, as levers for the purpose of removing irritation to the nervous system, which is the cause of a whole host of diseases, and called his system *chiropractic.* It has certain advantages over osteopathy and many osteopaths have either gone over to chiropractic, or combined the two types of therapy.

Papaya. A large green-skinned tropical fruit resembling a melon, with a fleshy peach-coloured interior containing dozens of black seeds, like round shot. When the fruit is cut in half these are

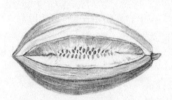

easily scooped out. The flesh is sweet and valued for its digestive *enzymes.* The juice is used in the East to soften meat before cooking, and render it easily digestible. The papaya is a good source of vitamin C. The fruit contains 76.60% water, 5.20% protein, 0.90% fat, 16.80% carbohydrates, and 0.50% mineral salts.

Peach. An excellent soft fruit introduced into Britain from Southern Europe and grown usually on south walls in sheltered gardens. It was thought that the peach would not flourish in exposed gardens till in 1936 a farmer in Suffolk planted 28 peach bushes on an exposed site 360

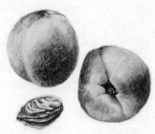

feet above sea level. He argued that they flourished in America and Canada where the climate is far more extreme than in Britain. His experiment exceeded all expectations and in due course he put down 50 acres of peach bushes, each of which produced hundreds of marketable peaches every year. A well ripened peach is a truly delicious fruit containing malic and citric acids and consisting of 88.10% water, 0.70% protein, 0.10% fat, 9.40% carbohydrates, and 0.40% mineral matter, mainly potassium. It also contains vitamins A, C and D, is a mild diuretic and good for dropsical, bladder and kidney diseases.

Pear. A succulent fruit but one of the most fickle of all as it is impossible to judge from its exterior whether it is fit to eat. One

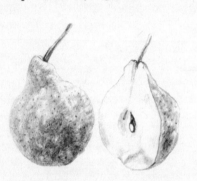

day it may be hard, the next ripe, on the third day over-ripe and on the fourth 'sleepy' and unpleasant. In the Middle Ages and for many years after so much over-ripe and rotten fruit was eaten, and conditions were so insanitary that diseases were often attributed to the eating of pears, and their popularity waned. The historian Matthew Paris says that pears were grown in Britain in 1257 but they were doubtless introduced much earlier. They were renowned for their flavour and cooling properties but not until recently for their alkalinity and vitamin content. They contain 84.00% water, 0.60% protein, 0.50% fat, 14.10% carbohydrates and 0.40% mineral matter, mainly potassium.

Phosphorus. A man weighing 150 lb has about 1 lb 14 oz of phosphorus in his body and though it is one of the principal constituents of the brain and, as Moleschott said 'there is no thought without phosphorus,' it does not follow that eating foods rich in this element will improve the brain power. Sea fish, pike and salmon are rich in phosphorus but eating them does not make one an intellectual. About 27 oz are contained in the bones, 2½ in the muscular tissues and 0.25 oz in the brain and nervous system.

Phosphorus, *calcium*, *sunlight* and *vitamin D* are necessary for growth, and if phosphorus is lacking the body withdraws some from the bones to make up this deficiency, just as it does when calcium is lacking. There are parts of the world, e.g. South Africa, where the soil is deficient in phosphorus and the result is seen in under-developed farm animals, which have to be given phosphorus supplements.

There is no need for anyone on a balanced diet to worry about his intake of phosphorus as milk, cheese, fish, oysters, beef, fruits dried and fresh, vegetables raw and cooked, contain small quantities and the sum total is sufficient to keep the body healthy.

Physiotherapy. Derived from the Greek *physio*, nature; and *therapeutikos*, to care, heal. A system of curing by massage, movements of the limbs and manipulation. It is quite distinct from *osteopathy* and *chiropractic*. *Chiropractic* deals mainly with adjustments to the spinal column which are designed to relieve tension on the nerves which radiate to every part of the body; and the *osteopath* adjusts the spine and breaks down lesions in various parts of the body. Physiotherapists deal mainly with sprains and strains in the limbs, neck, thorax and the abdominal region. Their range is more limited and though they have achieved success in cases of rheumatism and displaced bones they do not claim to cure a wide variety of diseases. They are recognised by the medical profession, can work only with the consent of doctors, and their services come within the NHS.

Pineapple. Why this fruit is called pineapple is unknown for like the custard-apple (a tropical fruit) and the love-apple (tomato) it bears not the slightest resemblance to the apple. It grows in the Southern States of America, South America, the West Indies, South Africa, India, Australia and Hawaii, not on a tree but on a

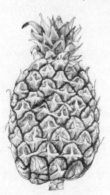

plant at ground level. It is a fickle fruit and must be harvested at a certain state; if left for a few days after ripening it loses piquancy and becomes flat and insipid. The pineapple has long been recognised in the tropics as a remedy for clearing the body of persistent mucous, and the juice is used not only to soften meat, but also corns and calluses. Recent analysis has revealed that it contains bromelain, the most remarkable of the proteolytic *enzymes*, which break down proteins into simpler and more assimilable

125

substances known as amino-acids. Bromelain has a soothing effect on pain and inflammation and when isolated has been known to relieve rheumatism and arthritis. Eating the whole fruit is preferable, however, for there are no side effects. The fruit is rich in malic acid and *vitamin C* and contains 89.30% water, 0.40% protein, 0.30% fat, 9.70% carbohydrates and 0.30% mineral matter, mainly potassium.

Plant Milk. A white viscous liquid obtained by processing grass, leaves and *beans* (soya in particular), having the colour and texture of milk and increasingly used by vegetarians and vegans and by people in the Third World who suffer from a lack of protein. Plant milk is made from the outer leaves of the cabbage, pea and pods and other greens, with B_{12} added, at the Vegetarian Nutritional Research Centre at Garston, Watford. The Centre is collaborating with the Food Research Centre in Coonoor, South India, established by *Dr Aykroyd* for producing edible products from leaves and grass. In one type of plant milk (Plamil) available in Britain the protein consists of 21 amino acids, including all the essential ones, and one pint contains 18 grammes of protein, and a pint of diluted (50/50) milk and water, 316 calories. It is available on the NHS on a doctor's prescription and is given to patients with lactose intolerance or a sensitivity to penicillin.

Plum. Grown for centuries in most English gardens. When ripe it is juicy with a full flavour and may be eaten either raw or stewed, and is one of the most popular fruit for making jams and fillings for pies and tarts. The original Christmas pudding contained plums, probably in the form of *prunes*. Plums contain a small amount of benzoic acid and the stones harbour a kernel which is rich in protein. Plums consist of 78.40% water, 1.00% protein, no fat, 20.00% carbohydrates and 0.60% mineral matter, mainly potassium.

Potassium. The body of a 150 lb man contains about 3 oz of potassium which exists in inorganic nature in the form of chloride and sulphate of potassium in sea water or in deposits of rock salt in the earth's crust. Seeds are rich in potassium, and phosphate of potassium is the mineral basis of all muscular tissues, endowing them with their characteristic pliancy.

Potassium salts play a part in forming glycogen from glucose, fats from glycogen, and proteins from peptones and proteoses. The liver contains twice as much potassium as *sodium* and the spleen a quarter. It is a predominant element in the red blood corpuscles and in the brain and is concerned in the generation of electricity in the body. Potassium and sodium have similar chemical properties but one cannot replace the other. All plants contain a good supply of potassium, dried fruit and nuts being particularly rich in this mineral, though almost everything we eat contains some and a deficiency of potassium is extremely rare.

Potato. A native of the Andes and the staple food of Indians living above the corn belt. Both the common potato and the sweet potato were cultivated extensively in Central and South America, where the Spanish discovered and called them *patata*, from which the English name is derived. It is an admirable 'filler', being cheap, bulky, tasty and capable of being concocted into a hundred different dishes. The Irish took to the potato with enthusiasm because it was easily grown, much hardier than wheat or barley, and occupied less space for an equivalent yield. In Britain it was resisted as an article of diet at first because rumour had it that potatoes caused leprosy and Cobbett said that the working man had more 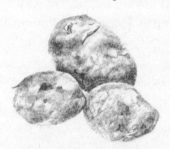 sense than to eat cattle food. The Scots did more than anyone to popularise it and by eating potatoes in their jackets from a cabman's stall, King Edward VII made the aristocracy follow his example.

There is no 'perfect food' but as an article of diet the potato has no peer. The scientist M. S. Rose existed in perfect health for four years exclusively on potatoes and milk and a number of other experimenters have lived for up to 300 days on potatoes and a little fat.

As old potatoes consist mainly of water (new potatoes contain the most starch), it is an ideal food for slimmers, provided the potato is not fried and little fat is eaten with it. It is easy to eat too much fat as the potato can absorb one fifth of its weight in fat without tasting too oily.

Potatoes vary in their composition, depending on whether they are old or new but within the limits of variation they contain 68-80% water, 0.69–3.70% protein, about 16.19% carbohydrates in the form of starch, 0.40–0.96% fat, 0.28–3.48% fibre and 0.53–1.87% mineral salts, mainly potassium. The potato baked in its jacket contains *vitamins A, B* and *C*. This is the best way to eat it for F. W. Price says in *Textbook of The Practice of Medicine* that 6 oz of potato daily, cooked for 15 minutes, will prevent scurvy. Boiling for longer destroys some of the vitamin C.

Preissnitz, Vincent (1791-1851). Started life tending sheep on the mountain side. He often watched deer and other injured animals limp down to the streams and immerse their limbs, sometimes for hours. They always moved off much improved, which convinced him that cold water, pure and simple, was a great healer. He tried out cold water on villagers with strains, bruises and broken limbs, with astonishing success. Then he treated other diseases, always with water at temperatures between 43° and 88°F – never warmer; but some considered his methods too harsh. He became renowned locally as a healer and would make serious invalids take ice-cold showers lasting from two to five minutes, in the open. After the *Sturzdusche* (torrent shower bath) they were given an air-and-water bath. Never did he resort to warm or hot water and though 40,000 patients passed through his hands only 45 deaths were registered, and those of patients given up by the medical profession. Though he also set much store on fresh air and exercise these were regarded as of secondary importance. Preissnitz might never have become famous had he not cured the Emperor when the royal physicians gave him up, and his reputation was so great that letters from America addressed to 'Herr Preissnitz, Europe', were invariably delivered. He also advised his patients about diet and told them to eat and drink in moderation.

His 'dripping sheet treatment' was renowned. In this a linen sheet was wrung out in cold water and placed over the shoulders of the patient, who was then rubbed energetically by assistants till his skin glowed and the sheet steamed. This drew blood to the surface of the skin and relieved internal organs. He used this treatment to cure diseases of the lungs, liver, heart, kidneys, brain – and also for cholera! But never for anaemia or nerves. Like *Kneipp*, he insisted that water treatment should never be administered except by an expert, otherwise harm rather than benefit might result. Preissnitz is generally regarded as the Father of *Hydrotherapy*. See: Hydrotherapy, Kneipp.

Preservatives in Food. More than 30 chemicals are used in Britain to preserve food, or to use the jargon in fashion 'give them a longer shelf-life'. Many chemicals are permitted because none are banned till proved (not suspected) dangerous to health. BHT (butylhydroxytolune) is one example. The *Australian Medical Journal* states that BHT in food given to mice resulted in 15% of them being born without eyes! West Germany banned it with one exception – it can be added to rations for the army; Sweden and Romania have banned it completely, yet the Ministry of Food in Britain is still considering the matter. In America the FDA* say that it is best left in the hands of 'the men with white jackets' (chemists). Wherever there is doubt about a preservative the lobby of the food and soft drinks industry, which has a strong interest for their use, brings pressure to bear on MPs to resist bans, irrespective of the harm they may do to health. All preservatives that are suspect should be banned till it has been proved they are not harmful. See: Processing, Saccharine.

Price Weston, MS, DDS, FACO. An American doctor and dental surgeon who travelled the world carrying out an investigation into the eating habits of people and to find out which foods gave health and which (or the lack of which) resulted in disease. He also investigated their habits, the climate in which they lived, their freedom from dental caries and degenerative diseases and their longevity, and the reasons for them. It was the first world-wide survey of its kind and the results, set out in *Nutrition and Physical Degeneration* have added considerably to our knowledge of dietetics and preventive medicine.

Processing Of Food. See: Chemicals in Food.

Proteins. Name given to a range of chemical substances used in the manufacture, in the body, of tissues and organs. Lean meat, for instance, consists of four different but similar proteins. They are among the essential substances which occur in animal and vegetable organisms, and protein metabolism is the most characteristic sign of life. All proteins consist of a number of building blocks called amino-acids; some are composed of only two or three; others as many as 20. They must be catabolised (broken down) in the body before they can be anabolised (built up) to form the natural proteins in the body, and this is done by ferments and *enzymes* in the digestive system.

*Food and Drug Administration.

Proteins

Plant proteins differ from animal proteins in the number and proportion of their constituent amino-acids, and those that lack the amino-acids essential to life are classed as 'second class proteins', and those that contain them as 'first class proteins'. Generally speaking vegetable proteins are considered to be 'second class' and those of meat and milk products 'first class'. But many vegetable proteins, when combined, provided first class proteins.

Amino-acids necessary for life are: valine, leucine, isoleucine, threonine, lysine, arginine, methionine, phenylalanine, tryptophan and histidine; there are doubts about glycine, and cystine is not essential. Some proteins, such as gelatine, are classed as 'complete' and 'good' but have very low nutritional value, whereas others from the vegetable kingdom such as nuts, legumes and beans, though classed as 'poor', have a high nutritional value, and if combined with other vegetable foods transform themselves in the body and perform the work of 'good' proteins. If this were not so it would be impossible to account for the health, strength and stamina of so many life-long vegetarians and vegans.

The tendency is to class meat and fish and milk products as 'first class' and beans, peas, nuts and legumes as 'second class'. *Sherman* says: 'In this case tradition has accumulated a strong prejudice which attributes superiority to 'animal protein' and inferiority to proteins of vegetable foods. This we know from modern research to be an unsound generalisation, yet this prejudice and prejudicial inheritance from a pre-scientific yesterday persists; and one so often meets the term 'animal protein' as part of a dietary description or specification in a way that plainly perpetuates the fallacy.

'Chemical research on the amino-acid constitution of animal proteins and nutrition research with human subjects in balance experiments and with laboratory animals over long segments of the life cycle (including the periods of rapid growth) rank the protein of *soya beans* and peanuts with animal proteins in chemical nature and nutritional efficiency; and show further that the proteins of our ordinary beans and peas need but little supplementation in order to nourish us equally well.'

Nuts and soya beans, says Sherman, have a higher biological value than legumes and 'roasted peanuts ground to peanut butter also make a highly nutritious and very convenient food. In a sandwich peanut butter fills the place of both butter and meat.' Nuts and legumes are a good source of *calcium* and *thiamine*.

Many sources of protein are as yet untapped. The Soviet scientist, Nikolai Turbin, has cultivated a newly evolved lupin, the seeds of which contain 42% protein, even more than the soya bean, which has many indispensable amino-acids. Ordinary lupin seeds should not be eaten as they are poisonous.

Prune. A dried plum, originally the main ingredient of the plum pudding, of plum porridge and the sugar plum, a crystalised prune. In the past 'mince meat' consisted of finely chopped ox-tongue, beef, suet, dried fruits and sugar; and plum pudding of tongue, spices, suet, bread crumbs, flour, wine, raisins, prunes and gravy.

Only certain varieties of dark plums are used to make prunes, which are dried either in the sun or artificially. With figs and beetroot they rate as the finest of natural aperients. On the Continent prunes are crystalised with marzipan and are used to soften the flavour of 'marc' brandy. Prune brandy is also made from the fruit. Prunes can be eaten with meat dishes, chopped up in salads, stuffed with cream cheese and used in a variety of ways. Prunes with boiled rice, a favourite in public schools in the past, is perhaps the most unimaginative way of serving them. The prune consists of 22.30% water, 2.20% protein, no fat, 71.20% carbohydrates, and 2.30% mineral matter, mainly potassium.

Psionic Medicine. Devised by Dr George Laurence, MRCS, LRCPL FRCS (Edin); is an extension of orthodox medicine and not an off-beat system of therapy. It depends on the existing body of medical and surgical experience. Where it differs from orthodox practice, however, is that the practitioner is trained to use perceptive sensitivity beyond the use of senses available through the five normal channels: sight, hearing, taste, touch and smell. Thus the prefix *psi*, adopted from the Greek letter to denote paranormal senses.

This added dimension which unfortunately eludes some practitioners, is used in the manipulation of the Abram's Box, the *de la Warr* system of radionics and diagnosis by the pendulum, used so successfully by Abbé Mermet and Dr Moineau. It is a sense not inherent in all and has to be developed.

Practitioners of Psionic Medicine maintain that though faulty diet, bad living conditions and infections play a significant part in disease, these are not the causes. They merely trigger off the physical and psychological symptoms to which the patient is predisposed constitutionally. The real causes which predispose the individual to illness, which homeopaths call *miasms*, may be inherited or are a hangover from some previous infection or a combination of both. When these *miasms* are eradicated, the symptoms, which indicate that something is wrong, disappear and the patient is cured; or in difficult cases, made more amenable to supportive treatment.

Allopathic medicine usually provides a rapid alleviation of distress and gives the body a chance to clear itself, for as Osler said, only Nature cures; the most the physician can do is to help Nature. Unfortunately, drugs which play so important a part in orthodox medicine today, often cause side effects, some extremely damaging. In Psionic Medicine, however, homeopathic remedies are used once the underlying causes of disease have been discovered, and there is no danger from side effects.

Because diagnosis by the pendulum enables practitioners to reveal the underlying causes of disease, they have achieved startling successes in the treatment of chronic and even 'incurable' diseases; and migraine, for instance, an affliction which causes unbelievable distress to tens of thousands in Britain alone, and has disrupted or ruined many lives, is frequently cured by this method. So, too, is asthma.

Psionic Medicine by J. H. Reyner in collaboration with George Laurence and Carl Upton, is a book which should be in the hands of all sufferers who have failed to gain relief from orthodox medicine.

The Psionic Medical Society, which is registered as a charity, trains doctors and dentists, instigates research and maintains a register of qualified practitioners. The address of the Institute of Psionic Medicine is: Beacon Hill Park, Hindhead, Surrey, GU26 6HU.

Pulse. Edible seeds of leguminous plants such as beans, peas, and *lentils*. *McCarrison*, who carried out experiments between 1929 and 1934 in India with 1,000 rats, said: 'If man did not provide in his own person the proof that a diet composed of whole cereal grains, or a mixture of certain grains, milk, milk-products, pulses and fresh vegetables, with meat occasionally, sufficed for optimum physical efficiency, this experience in rats would do so.' Pulses form the staple food of many under-developed nations and should be eaten far more widely in the rice-eating countries as they would form a valuable supplement to their diet. See: Legumes, Beans, Lentils.

Pumpkin. Originally called pumpion for the word was derived from the Greek *pepon*, meaning cooked in the sun. It is a gourd and a native of India and Africa but now grown in almost every country in the world. In the tropics it is valued for its cooling properties for it contains 90.30% water, 1.10% protein, 0.13% fat, 6.50% carbohydrates and 0.70% mineral matter, mainly potassium, sodium and phosphorus. In India the seeds have been used in *ayurvedic* medicine for centuries for urinary disorders and expelling tape worms. Sometimes the flesh is used as a substitute for the seeds. Potter's *New Encyclopedica of Botanical Drugs and Preparations* also recommends the seeds, beaten into a paste, for expelling tape worms. Since the war research on folk remedies has discovered that pumpkin seeds have a powerful effect on the prostate gland, which in males past the age of 50 has a tendency to become enlarged due to the organ's efforts to compensate for the loss of male hormones, which start to decline. Ancient Hindus used it as a cure for prostate troubles and their lore was carried by gypsies to Turkey, Hungary and the Ukraine. The seeds are richer in *phosphorus* and *iron* than any other seeds, and contain *vitamins A* and *B*.

Purgatives. What Hippocrates wrote in *Prognostics* more than 2,000 years ago remains true today; that evacuation should take place twice or thrice a day and once at night, in proportion to the food eaten. Constipation is a modern disease and a curse of civilisation. It used to be called 'the American Disease' but with the adoption of so many of America's eating habits, especially their pappy breakfast foods, it is now also 'the English disease', and a vast quantity of laxatives in the form of pills and liquid oils are swallowed by millions. For many a laxative each morning is as necessary as a cup of tea and there are thousands who do not have a bowel movement more than *once a week*, and some patients are even told by their doctors that a bowel movement every day is not necessary!

There are many reasons for constipation, the most common of all diseases: (1) the bolting of food without adequate mastication

(2) the pappy foods which do not need mastication (3) denatured and processed foods (4) excessive eating of refined starchy foods (5) flabby stomach muscles (6) lack of exercise.

A purgative such as Glauber Salts should be taken only when the bowels fail to act, followed by a short fast of about three days, after which the diet should be regulated by eating plenty of salads, nuts, fresh and dried fruit – especially beetroot, prunes and figs. All white flour products should be replaced by wholewheat, and bran should be sprinkled over soup, porridge and even salads to provide roughage and additional B1. Osteopathy and chiropractic treatment will also help. See: Bran, Constipation, Diverticulitis.

Pyridoxine. See: Vitamin B6.

Q

Quack. According to the Oxford English Dictionary 'An ignorant pretender to medical skill; one who boasts to have a knowledge of wonderful remedies; an empiric or imposter in medicine.' The word is used disparagingly by allopaths to describe practitioners of any other form of healing; in fact, anyone who does not subscribe to the orthodox view. *naturopaths, herbalists,* bone-setters, *chiropractors, osteopaths, acupuncturists,* etc.

Words often change their meanings with the passage of time and today the word 'quack', which once described a barker at a fair who prescribed pills and potions, has taken on a different meaning, and one often hears the question put to patients after a visit to the doctor: 'And what did the quack have to say?' This may be because unorthodox healers are having so much success and are curing thousands who have failed to gain relief at the hands of their NHS doctors. The sooner orthodox medicine realises its limitations and works in conjunction with other therapies, the better will it be for the health of the nation.

R

Race and Food. Food reformers often become cranky in their outlook or grow so rabid that they imagine that they alone know all the answers, and allow no latitude to those who fail to fall into line. New converts to a regimen are among the worst. They close their eyes to the fact that there are many kinds of widely diverging diets in the world on which men have lived in perfect health for generations. There is, in fact, no ideal diet for all. The Scots in the past lived mainly on oats, barley and herrings, a diet that supplied the nourishment needed in that northern clime. The Russians eat excessive amounts of fat to combat their bone-crushing cold; so do the Tibetans, who add barley and rancid butter to tea and boil the lot; and Eskimos seem to thrive on blubber, seal meat (often putrid), lichens and tallow candles. A Captain Gray describes how Australian Aborigines danced and shrieked with joy when a rotting whale was washed ashore. 'They rubbed the blubber over their naked bodies,' he relates, 'and those of their favourite wives; after which they opened a passage through the whale's fat down to the lean meat..... you could see them climbing over the stinking carcase in search of more delicate morsels....' In the South Seas masses of worms are regarded as delicacies at certain times of the year, and almost anything that can be masticated is found to be edible – and good – in some part of the world. 'The Sandy Lake Indians,' according to C. C. and S. M. Furnas, 'boiled the excrement of rabbits with their rice to season it.' Tasmanian aborigines use ashes to season and spice their food, and an American painter who lived among them said that some Indian tribes subsisted by eating about a pound of dirt (earth) a day.

Generally speaking, their natural habitat produces the food best suited to those who live in it. Curries, for instance, are eaten throughout the East because food putrifies easily in torrid zones and is prevented from doing so by spices, which are powerful preservatives and contain essential minerals and vitamins.

Too sudden a change from one traditional diet to another wholly dissimilar often leads to a breakdown in health, though Man can be weaned gradually from one kind of diet to another. With the growth of communications and the swift rate of travel the eating habits of most civilised communities are undergoing a gradual change. A prime example is Britain where the traditional breakfast was bacon and eggs, kidney, liver and sausage, porridge, marmalade and toast, and tea or coffee. This has been supplanted largely by patent breakfast foods; and heavy meals of beef and other meats have given way to salads and fruit; and instead of ale which the Elizabethans had for breakfast, almost everyone drinks tea.

People should not be dogmatic and insist that because certain foods suit them they will agree with everyone else. There was a small group of farmers in the corn belt of the Mid-West of America who seemed to keep excellent health mainly on a diet of onions and whisky; and when I was a young man living in 'digs' I often supped off a whole cucumber and coffee, which in no way affected my slumbers or digestion. I know one old lady who often said to me: 'Coffee always sends me to sleep', though it doesn't have that effect on most people. See: Smell, Taste, Tongue.

Radiesthesia. The art of detecting and diagnosing disease by passing hands over the body, based on the theory that disease comes from a disturbance of the balance of energy radiating from the organic cells and that the wave lengths of radiations emitted from the body change during disease. Some practitioners use a pendulum instead of hands and a few, such as Abbé Mermet and Dr Moineau claim to be able to cure disease diagnosed under these conditions. Dr Moineau has used the pendulum to diagnose pregnancy as early as the first week of conception, and Abbé Mermet claims that he can state precisely which organ is diseased. Some sceptics call it 'scientific clairvoyance'. See: Psionic medicine.

Radionics. Often confused with *radiesthesia*. It is based on the same theory but does not depend on clairvoyance. Radionics is a science which deals instrumentally with the radiations of all forms of matter but more especially with human radiations. It can be applied to diagnose and treat disease by physical irradiation or distant radiation. It should be clearly understood, however, that radionic diagnosis is not a diagnosis of the physical body and should not be interpreted in the physical sense. Apparatus has been evolved to use the thought of the skilled operator as a probe in determining the basic causes of ill-health, even if they be psychological in origins. The same procedure can be applied in the diagnosis and treatment of trees, plants and crops, whether on a small or large scale.

An electrical instrument containing a number of magnetic coils is used, which tunes into the emitted vibrations, enabling the disease to be detected and diagnosed. Then vibrations are sent out by the machine which alleviate or cure, often over considerable distance – sometimes thousands of miles. Goethe was the first to propound the theory, followed by Reichenbach, who named life-radiation OD (odic force). The American pioneer was Dr Abrams, whose work was carried out by Ruth

Drown. Dr W. E. Boyd in Glasgow and Dr Guyon Richards in London were the medical pioneers in Britain, but no one did more work in this field than George de la Warr, who first studied homeopathy and then turned to acoustic therapy and finally to radiesthesia and radionics. Today radionics is accepted by the medical profession and many physicians collaborate with practitioners at the de la Warr Laboratories and elsewhere in Britain.

Raisin. The raisin is a grape partially dried either in the sun or artificially, like the sultana, currant, *fig* and *date*. It is a concentrated food high in calorific value but containing very little fat. It is valuable because it deteriorates very slowly, can be easily packed and carried and in combination with either nuts or fresh fruit can serve as an adequate substitute for a meal. Hikers, for instance, can sustain themselves for a long time on nuts and raisins. They contain 14.60% water, 2.60% protein, 3.30% fat, 73.60% carbohydrates and 3.40% mineral matter, mainly potassium and phosphorus. These values differ slightly, depending on the variety of grape dried.

Raw Food. Theoretically, uncooked foods are superior to cooked because they retain all the minerals and vitamins, and hard foods such as nuts, raw carrots and apples clean the surface of the teeth by removing particles of food and so help to preserve the enamel. Raw foods also exercise the gums and keep them healthy. But they need to be ground down to a pulp before being swallowed, otherwise they are liable to be indigestible. Those who have lived on cooked foods should not change suddenly but should gradually insert a little more raw food into their diet each week. A sudden transition may upset the system; moreover, there are millions equipped with dentures who find it difficult to deal with raw food, especially the harder or more stringy kinds of vegetables, such as celery; and of course, fruit such as figs and raspberries are anathema to this group. But even people with dentures can deal with most types of raw food if they cut them into small pieces, for often the cutting teeth do not have enough leverage to bite into apples or carrots and become displaced if pressure is placed on them.

Cooked foods have become part of civilised life and there are edibles such as bread, cakes and biscuits which cannot be eliminated from normal diet; and many vegetables cannot be eaten raw. During summer and autumn when fresh fruit and vegetables abound. 75% of the diet should consist of raw food, provided it can be chewed without discomfort and does not upset the digestion. Food is meant not only for nourishment but to be enjoyed and there is no point in being a martyr. When vegetables are cooked they should be steamed or casseroled and the liquid used as stock. They should not be boiled to death and soda should never be used to 'bring out the colour' in greens. It destroys *vitamin C* and is the cause of much indigestion. Prolonged use can lead to stomach ulcers. In all things let commonsense be your guide and avoid faddists.

Reich, Dr Wilhelm (1879-1957).American scientist and psychoanalyst who discovered a new kind of energy akin to static electricity, with healing power, which he labelled orgone. He was an early collaborator with Freud. Orgone is bluish in colour, emanates from the sun and affects all living organs. Clouds and bodies of water accumulate and store it and it is the best guarantee of health. Reich made blankets consisting of layers of inorganic and organic material containing orgone, which he claimed prevented and cured colds, rheumatism, arthritis and even polio. Though more than 80% of his patients were cured he was hounded by the American Medical Association, prosecuted under the Pure Foods and Drugs Act and, when he refused to curb his activities, was jailed. He committed suicide in prison. He wrote 30 books including *Orgone Accumulator, The Cancer Biopathy*, etc., and today many of his theories have been accepted and his name vindicated.

Reichenbach, Baron Karl Von (1788-1869). German industrial chemist famous for extracting paraffin and creosote from wood tar, and for numerous experiments on human subjects. He found that some highly sensitive people felt a cool stream of air near the north pole of a magnet, and in a darkened room could distinguish a bluish vapour or flame; and from the south pole a warm stream and an orange colour. This phenomenon was not confined to magnets but applied also to rock crystal as well. Many other substances were seen to emit colours and if his subjects remained in a dark room for two or three hours they could detect a glow of light from plants and animals.

Reichenbach said that in addition to white light the sun, moon and planets emitted an emanation which he called Od, Odyle or Odic Force which was distinct from electricity, magnetism and other forms of radiation. He named this force after the ancient Norse god Odin who was supposed to rule all nature. His experiments were confirmed by De Roches, the famous French hypnotist and psychic investigator and William Gregory, Professor of Chemistry at Edinburgh University.

Rheumatism. More than 8,000,000 a year seek medical help for some form of rheumatic complaint and in Britain in 1977 more than 44,000,000 working days were lost through the disease, 140,000 were confined to their homes, 50,000 to wheelchairs and beds and among them were 12,000 children. Though it is the most wide-spread of all degenerative diseases in Britain, Dr Philip Wood, author of *Rheumatism: The Price We Pay* says: 'The majority of GPs have no reasonable training in the diagnosis and treatment of rheumatism and arthritis. We have efficacious methods of treating patients, but they are not effectively employed.' Rheumatism is usually caused by damp living conditions and a lack of sunshine and there are people who have suffered for years and then, on retirement to Italy or Spain have found that suddenly their aches and twinges have vanished. The wrong *diet* is, of course, a prime cause and when this has been revised and vitamins C, D and E have been taken sufferers have been cured or any any rate, relieved. *Fasting* before a change of diet makes the chances of a cure much greater. *Acupuncture, naturotherapy, herbal treatment, homeopathy, chiropractic, osteopathy, hydrotherapy* and *ultra-violet ray* treatment have all been effective in curing patients after they have tried the round of specialists and hospitals. Many a rheumatic sufferer has improved by doing naught else but substituting whole wheat products for white, and cutting out all white sugar. In 1948 Captain Oliver Bird, head of the famous custard firm, who was a martyr to rheumatism donated £450,000 towards research into the disease, but it did not bring him relief. Lord Horder described rheumatism as Public Enemy No. 1, and today Britain spends £400,000 a year in rheumatism relief –mainly 'wonder-drugs' which bring in their train disastrous side-effects, and other systems which are curing hundreds of rheumatic sufferers every year, are ignored. Lord Horder said: 'Rheumatic disease in most of its forms is not curable by a bottle of medicine for internal use and a linament for external use.' *Nettles* and *pustulants* often cure when orthodox medicine fails.

Riboflavin. See: Vitamin B2.

Rice: Polished and Brown. The rice sold in most supermarkets and grocers' shops is white or polished rice; that sold in health food stores and shops that sell Indian spices is 'brown' rice, which is much darker and sometimes covered by a reddish-brown skin. This is the pericarp, which may be dullish-white, yellow, rust-coloured or even nearly black – or any combination of these colours. It is this coating, just under the husk, which contains the essential vitamin B_1.

Polished rice, much whiter in colour, is the result of further milling, has much lower food value, and is mainly carbohydrate in the form of starch. In 1897 Eijkman, a Dutch doctor in Java, observed that fowls fed on white rice developed polyneuritis and when given rice with the reddish skin on it, recovered rapidly. Other experiments proved the value of this outer covering, and years later McCarrison showed that prolonged washing of brown rice removed this outer coating. The idea that rice should be washed again and again before being cooked, is wrong. It doesn't get any cleaner. After the First World War *Osler* and Viscount Bryce used their influence to persuade the British Government to impose a heavy tax on polished rice, but progress of the Bill through Parliament was so slow that both died before aught was accomplished.

Rikli, Arnold (1823-1906). Founder of the modern sun-and-air cure. The Greeks and Romans believed that exposure to sunlight and fresh air hardened the body and made it resistant to disease. In the Middle Ages when the cult of dirt was followed assiduously by the best people, their ideas fell into disuse. Between 1750-1850 the Germans Hufeland, Leobel, Doberereiner and Rosenbaum, and the Frenchmen Bonnet and Lebert cured leg ulcers, rickets, scrofula and tuberculosis of the bones and joints by exposure to fresh air and sun. The chief apostle, however, was Rikli of Wagen on the Aare, a Swiss, who established the first sanatorium for fresh air and sun treatment in Veldes in Oberkrain (today a part of Yugoslavia). Dr Heinrich Lahmann was one of his most important disciples and introduced Rikli's treatment into his world-famous sanatorium, Weissen Hirsch (White Hart) near Dresden. From 1900 fresh-air-and-sun cures in the Engadin, especially Davos, became world famous for the treatment of TB. Dr Rollier started his treatment along the same lines, for tuberculosis of the glands, bones and joints at Leysin.

Rikli believed also in hydrotherapy and a reformed diet but stated: 'Water may well do it, but air is better; but light is best of all.' His patients lived in specially designed 'air huts', and bare feet were compulsory; but he also set high value on the healing power of warmth and fevers produced by artificial heat. The *skin*, he maintained, was the most important of all organs and he advocated sweat-baths and vigorous exercise to rid the body of poisons.

He said: 'A full supply of fresh air – pure air – is of the utmost importance for the cure of all diseases, be it a cold or typhoid or cholera, rheumatism or gout, nervousness or consumption, cancer or syphilis, a wound or an open sore;' and Dr Lahman added: 'The open sleeping rooms, the air huts invented by Rikli, are a benefit to sufferers from lung disease, sleeplessness and poverty of the blood, which cannot be sufficiently extolled.'

He was a picturesque figure resembling an old-world prophet, with leather shorts and bare legs, who strode hundreds of miles through Austria and Germany, preaching his sermons on health and gathering converts wherever he went. He slept with wide-open windows in the coldest weather and never suffered a day's illness.

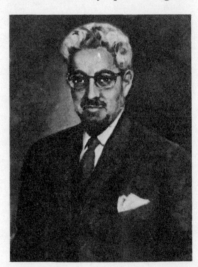

J. I. Rodale

Rodale, J. I. (1899-1971). An apostle of health foods and a pioneer of organic gardening in America, who for years was criticised by the establishment for saying: 'The world is a biological organism, not a chemical laboratory,' a truth which has now sunk in and been accepted by scientists.

An accountant by training, he had an urge to educate and became publisher of a number of digests, the best known being *The Fact Digest* which had a circulation of 100,000. Among his magazines were two on health for he was a disciple of the English agronomist, *Sir Albert Howard*. Although not a farmer he learnt all about growing food by the organic method and started an Organic Gardening Experimental Farm near Allentown, Penn. in 1942, which eventually became a show place visited by people from every state in America and from continents abroad. For 30 years no chemical fertiliser or pesticide was used. Then, as he believed that prevention is better than cure, he founded the health magazine *Prevention* to propagate organic farming methods and other health ideas, and to warn against additives, processed foods, detergents and harmful sprays, long before the medical profession or any government body did so. He died in harness, giving a talk on health to a TV audience, but his ideas live on.

Rollier, Dr. A disciple of *Finsen*, who learnt from Yanowsky that sunlight has the power to kill typhoid bacteria, and from Downes and Blunt that it killed other germs as well. Finsen died prematurely but Rollier followed the work of *Rikli* at his nature cure home at Valdes where patients benefited by his *'cure atmospherique'*, and in 1903 started his world-famous clinic at Leysin where sunlight was used all the year round. He in turn inspired Sir Henry Gauvain, who established a sun-cure home at Alton and his methods were taken up by Queen Mary's Hospital in Carshalton, Guy's Hospital and other teaching hospitals in London. Rollier was, however, the pioneer of sun and ultra-violet treatment, and he said 'Sun and ultra-violet rays bear much the same relation to one another as crude drugs do to their synthetically prepared chemical substitutes.' Later Rollier revised many of his ideas and to a large extent practised naturopathy in conjunction with sun and ultra-violet ray treatment. He had phenomenal success in treating tuberculosis of the glands, bones and joints as well as pulmonary tuberculosis. When Dr. Bernhard Detmar, the famous German physician visited Leysin and expressed astonishment at the remarkable physical condition of the patients, and said: 'How is it possible that these patients who have to remain lying the whole time and can only work a little, if indeed at all – how is it that they have such powerful muscles?' To which Rollier replied: 'The sun does it all – just the sun.' Though Rollier is dead his clinic at Leysin is still carried on by those whom he taught and who taught others.

Rontgen, (pronounced Runtghen), **Wilhelm Konrad** (1845-1923). Born in Lennep, Germany; studied mechanical engineering at Zurich, was recognised as one of the foremost experimental physicists of his day and held a number of important appointments at several German universities. In 1895 while studying an electrical discharge produced in a vacuum tube he noticed that a piece of paper nearby which had been coated with barium platinocyanide, was fluorescing brilliantly. He covered it with a black card but it continued to fluoresce and within a few weeks he proved that this was caused by an invisible ray, which though not seen by the human eye passed easily through paper and wood, but not metal and other dense materials. This was called the Rontgen Ray but for simplification is now known as the X-ray and his discovery earned him the Nobel Prize for Physics in 1901.

Rontgen-Rays. or **X-rays.** Electromagnetic waves of the same type as light but of much shorter wave length, produced when cathode rays (a stream of electrons) strike a material object. X-rays affect a photographic plate in a way similar to that of light. The absorption of the rays by matter depends upon the density and the atomic weights of the materials. The lower the AW and density, the more transparent the material is to X-rays. Thus, bones being more opaque than the surrounding flesh make it possible to take an X-ray photograph of the skeleton of a living person. This is invaluable in the treatment of patients by *osteopathy, chiropractic* and by the medical profession for intestinal diseases and fractures.

Root Vegetables. Included in this category are bulbs, roots and tubers: Jerusalem artichokes, beets, *carrots,* parsnips,

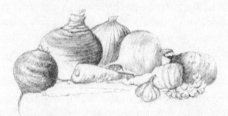

swedes, mangolds, *potatoes,* salsify, *onions* and *garlic.* All these plants store sugar and starches in roots and underground stems; sometimes, as in the onion family, in swollen modified leaves. Root vegetables are excellent fillers, a good source of energy, and the roughage they contain assists bowel movement.

Rutin. It is known that the vitamins *C, K, P, B*12 and *folic acid* assist the free flow of blood through the arteries and capillaries, the tiny hair-like vessels which bring blood into contact with the tissues. Vitamin K concerns the clotting of blood; folic acid and B12 are concerned with the health of red blood corpuscles; vitamin C (ascorbic acid) has many functions, one being the prevention of tissue bleeding, and another the maintenance of the state of equilibrium between the fluid plasma in the capillaries and the fluid in the tissues of the heart and circulation.

Within the past 50 years two other substances which affect the circulation have been discovered: citrin, a composition of several compounds known as glucosides, the best known of which is hesperidin; and another glucoside called rutin, which is found in many plants, among them elderflowers, violets, forsythia, and the leaves and flowers of buckwheat. When analysed the leaves and flowers of buckwheat were found to contain 4% of rutin on a dry weight basis. Experiments carried out in Britain, America and the Continent prove that a tea made from rutin is effective in the treatment of hypertension, vascular disorders, coronary occlusion and apoplexy.

S

Saccharin (benzoic sulphamide). Discovered by Dr Remsen who was awarded a medal by the American Chemical Society for his achievement. In 1902 Dr Harvey W. Wiley, Chief of the Bureau of Chemistry in the Department of Agriculture, USA, formed a 'poison squad' of volunteers to investigate the adulteration of food, such as alum in baking powder, benzoate of soda in catsup and sulphate of copper in peas and green vegetables to preserve their colour. All three and many others were banned. Then he turned his attention to saccharin, which he and his squad found to be harmful if taken over a protracted period. But when they recommended that it should be banned, the 'saccharin lobby' headed by Congressman J. S. Sherman (later Vice-President of the USA) appealed to the President, who appointed a board under Dr Remsen (!) to report on the matter. It happened that the President (Theodore Roosevelt) had been advised by Dr Rixey to take saccharin instead of sugar to keep down his weight, so when the Remsen Board declared in its favour he refused to ban the drug.

Two further attempts were made to ban other drugs, among them saccharin, in 1906 and 1912 but though the law stated that it was a deleterious substance and the substitution of saccharin for sugar in foods lowers their quality, it was not banned in America till the 9th March 1977 when both the FDA and the Canadian government said that their scientists believed it caused cancer in laboratory animals. See: Wiley.

Salads. Most people imagine that the custom of serving salads is a recent one because during the past half century the usual salad served in most British restaurants consisted of a lettuce leaf and a few slices of tomato and cucumber. Two or three hundred

years ago fresh garden vegetables as we know them did not exist
in Britain and had to be imported at considerable cost. Only the
rich could afford them. Country folk scoured the fields and
woods and hedgerows for dandelions, nettles, dill, salsify, sorrel, dock, watercress, collards, garlic, onions, mint, parsley,
sage, coltsfoot, scurvey-root, camomile, elderflowers, mar-
joram, borage, fennel, tansy, wormwood, horehound, balm
and similar herbs. Sage, for instance, was first known as 'salvia',
meaning health, and then 'sage' meaning wise, for an old saying
runs: 'He who would live for aye, must eat sage in May.'

These and modern vegetables are good for the blood; the old
ones even more so because they are usually far more deep-
rooted and their roots break up and draw minerals from the
earth which shallow-roots fail to do. A salad should always
accompany or follow a dish in which the main ingredients are
protein, whether meat, fish, cheese or nuts, for salads are
alkaline and help to maintain a correct balance of the blood.

Salt (Sodium Chloride). Despite the commonly held belief that
salt is necessary for life, this is not so. We are told that animals in
their natural state often search for 'salt licks' and burrow for salt,
but they do so only when the herbiage on which they feed is
lacking in salt through soil erosion or leaching. Men who do
heavy work in steel mills and foundries where the heat is excessive are given saltwater to replace the salt they lose by excessive
sweating. Nature never intended man to work so hard in such
unnatural conditions, and unnatural conditions demand an
unnatural remedy. If you live on a balanced diet salt is unnecessary for fruit and vegetables contain all the minerals needed for
health. To test this you need only put a stick or two of celery
through an electric juicer and sample the juice, which will seem
inordinately salty.

The use of salt is by no means universal. When America was
discovered the settlers found that the Indians did not add salt to
their food; the Eskimos abhor salt and millions in Central Africa
never used any in food till it was introduced by Europeans. It
aggravates many diseases, chiefly those of the heart and circulation and excessive salt causes hypertension. It is one of the worst
enemies of sleep. Dr Michael Miller, associate physician of St.
Elizabeth's Hospital, Washington, D.C. conducted a simple
experiment a few years ago on people who could not sleep, by
reducing their intake of salt to 0.5 grammes a day. Twenty
patients, all suffering from insomnia took part. All were highly

tense, one in such a state that he could not concentrate in order to read; three others suffered from racking headaches. After a week on this almost salt-free diet the worst sufferers were able to sleep for 15 minutes and by degrees most of them responded in the most amazing way.

Professor Coirault, head of the Neuro-psychiatric Department of the biggest military hospital in France, says that when too much salt is taken the body cells work overtime to eject the surplus; this they do normally at night when the body is at rest. After conducting hundreds of experiments with patients he found that if given large quantities of salt with their evening meal they would lie awake till the small hours or even indulge in sleep walking and when eventually they fell asleep their slumbers were fitful and spasmodic. When given food completely free of salt they slept deeply and peacefully. The body needs about 5 grammes of salts a day, which can be obtained from natural sources; yet most people eat from 10 to 30 grammes of sodium chloride a day in addition to this.

Dr Flanders Dunbar states in *Mind and Body: Psychosomatic Medicine*, that salt is an important factor in migraine. Pressure is set up in the cranium by an increased flow of water to the blood vessels; but when placed on a salt-free diet relief in most cases is instantaneous.

I have not added salt to anything I've eaten for 50 years and reject the idea that 'salt brings out the flavour in food'. What it does is to mask the real taste of foods. It is the enemy of skin diseases and Ferdinand Sauerbruch, the famous German surgeon, cured many cases of skin irritation, and lupus, by placing patients on an entirely salt-free diet.

The Gentleman's Magazine of 6th September 1734 records that 'In France died the Sieur Michael Tourant, aged 98, of whom it is said that he never ate salt, and had none of the infirmities of old age.'

Sandow, Eugene. During the first 40 years of this century the name Sandow was synonymous with great physical strength, though in his youth he was sickly and weak and always in bed with some childish complaint. When he contracted tuberculosis the family doctor told his parents he would not last long, but Sandow had other ideas. He was intelligent and applied himself to the study of the body and realised that good food, fresh air and exercise which made him sweat profusely every day was the way to health. He became a member of the local *Ling* association

and practised free
movements but they did
not build up the strength he
craved for; so he took up
acrobatics and coupled them
with heavy work with
dumb-bells and bar bells.

He invented spring
dumb-bells which had to
be gripped tightly while
exercising, and the chest
expander, and started a
gymnasium in St. James's
Street, London, where he
turned weaklings into
powerful men. His system
consisted of resistance
exercises and deep breathing
and he claimed that he could

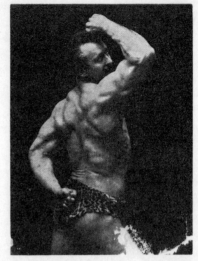

Eugene Sandow

put six inches on a normal man's chest in six months. His
exercises were founded on a knowledge of the body for he had
been a medical student. Thousands of men and *women* from all
over Britain flocked to him and thousands more who could not
make the journey wrote, asking his advice. So he started a
correspondence course, which he sold with his dumb-bells and
chest expanders. Soon he had pupils from every corner of the
British Empire and his name became a household one. He did an
enormous amount of good and brought health and strength to
hundreds of thousands. Many of the working classes who were
under-nourished and puny and failed the physical test for the
Army, went to Sandow's gymnasium, increased their chest
measurements and were accepted. During the First World War
he advised the authorities on physical fitness. Since his day
there have been men far bigger and much stronger but none has
captured the imagination of the public as Sandow did, nor put
their knowledge into practice so effectively.

Sauna Bath. A Finnish custom. The room in which the bath is
taken contains a stove heated by a wood fire. Water is sprinkled
on stones surrounding the stove, causing steam to rise and the
heat generated may be as much as 190°F. Usually there are three
steps along one side of the 'hot' room, the temperature on the
top step being greater than at floor level. When the body has

been thoroughly heated the bather is beaten with *vihta,* bunches of green twigs cut from the birch early in summer when the leaves are young and soft. The *vihta* is always softened in hot water each time before it is used. The beating increases the circulation but the idea that the sauna is a rejuvenating process is nonsense. After being beaten the bather is dipped in a lake or stream, and in winter rolled in the snow. The sauna toughens the body and enables it to resist the cold, which in Finland is intense, but it is no better than a warm bath or shower followed by a cold one and a brisk rub-down. The almost magical claims for the sauna are born in the heads of advertising men. In Britain the steam for saunas is produced electrically and not by sprinkling water on heated stones, and the effect is much the same as that of the Turkish bath. See: Bathing.

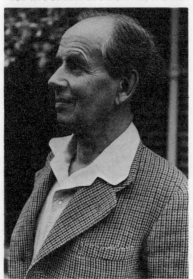

Edgar Saxon

Saxon, Edgar (1878-1956). Descended from Suffolk farmers and Cornish folk, who entered journalism by writing advertisements for the *British Weekly* in 1903, and eventually founded *Health and Life,* for many years the foremost vegetarian journal in Britain. Among the contributors were world famous figures such as GBS, the *Kelloggs,* Dr Valentine Knaggs, Dion Byngham and Henry Salt. The magazine was noted for its sane outlook and tolerance towards those who did not subscribe to its ideas. Saxon was the first to insist on the one-ness of Nature and believed in conservation. Most *vegetarians* in his day – because they were outcasts – were rabid and cranky and drunk with self-righteousness. Many practised self-immolation, but Saxon believed in enjoying the good things in life: music, food and wine. He believed in the inter-dependency of the human, animal, vegetable and mineral worlds. He saw, long before most people, that the preservation of the environment was essential to Man's advancement and survival. When he ceased to edit the journal Britain was the poorer, for it was a sane, well balanced magazine uninfluenced by the power of money or advertising. He lectured widely, wrote hundreds of articles on health and food reform, as well as poetry and some of his books – *A Sense of Wonder, Sensible Food For All*, and *Why Aluminium Pans Are Dangerous* – are still available.

Schussler, Dr Wilhelm Heinrich. Born in Oldenburgh, Germany; founder of the Biochemic system of medicine.

Schussler Biochemic System of Medicine. Biochemic medicine is based on the physiological fact that both the structure and vitality of the organs are dependent on certain essential inorganic salts in proper proportions. Schussler said: 'The inorganic substances in

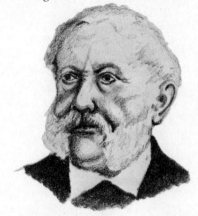

Dr W. H. Schussler

the blood and tissues are sufficient to heal all diseases which are curable. The question whether this or that disease is or is not dependent on the existence of fungi, germs or bacilli, is of no importance in biochemic treatment. If the remedies are used according to the symptoms, the desired end, that of curing diseases, which have been brought on by over-dosing, excessive use of medicines such as quinine, mercury, etc., can be cured by minute doses of cell-salts.' Biochemic salts are used by *homeopaths* and, though the system was devised long before the discovery of *vitamins* it is still as effective today as in Schussler's time.

The essential salts are: (1) Cf or Calcar Fluor (2) Cp or Calcar Phos (3) Cs or Calcar Sulph (4) Fp or Ferrum Phos (5) Km or Kali Mur (6) Kp or Kali Phos (7) Ks or Kali Sulph (8) Mp or Magnesia Phos (9) Nm or Natrum Mur (10) Np or Natrum Phos (11) Ns of Natrum Sulph (12) S or Silicea.

Scroth Cure Diet. Johann Scroth was an Austrian who founded a Nature Cure establishment in Lindewiesse, where he had tremendous success in curing gout, scrofula, swelling of the glands, skin diseases and even syphilis by his Dry Diet. His theory was that in every diseased condition fever was a curative factor and a necessary consequence of the health strivings of Nature. He maintained that no disease could be radically removed unless a sufficiently strong temperature could be raised. The fever purified the blood and juices from the contaminating matters of disease were removed through the pores of the skin.

(1) For the first three days patients were given no liquids and only stale white bread or rolls to eat, which acted like a sponge and absorbed poisons and mucous. (2) This was followed by two days of partial thirst and then a meal consisting of boiled rice, semolina, pearl barley, millet, and macaroni with lemon juice, but without fat of any sort. Also oatmeal gruel and lemon juice and an evening meal of bread with a small quantity of red or white wine. (3) Then two drink days; bread and oatmeal gruel and a little white wine in the evening. In the middle of the day stews as usual. The diet was modified to suit the idiosyncrasies of patients.

During the 'thirst' days the patient was covered by wet sheet packs, the skin greedily absorbing the moisture in the packs, assuaging thirst, and the warmth generated dissolved and excreted the matter of disease. After his death Scroth's son carried on the establishment till the 1914 war. His diet brought health to thousands whom the doctors could not cure and saved many from surgical operations. Apparently there are still many who pin their faith in the Scroth Dry Diet for when I visited Georges Hackenschmidt, former world champion wrestler in his home in South London (he was then past 80 but still instructing the police in the art) about 30 years ago, he was undertaking a 'dry fast' as advocated by Scroth.

Seaweed. Seaweed has been eaten for centuries in various forms in different parts of the world, by people living in coastal regions. If has also been ploughed into the soil to increase fertility. There are many varieties of seaweed: dulse, kelp, agar-agar, etc. Today it is used widely to make jellies, thicken soups and sauces, as a filler in cakes, ice-cream and other foods; and industrially in many forms. Most tooth-pastes, for instance, have a seaweed base. The oceans contain inexhaustible stores of weed, some growing to immense size, up to 700 feet long. Plants off the shores of San Clemente Island between Redondo and San Pedro Breakwater, are so large that a single specimen may contain as much as three tons of iodine worth as much as

£10,000. In America kelp farming is controlled by the government which decrees that no more than three feet may be sheared off the top of each bed, leaving the roots intact.

Seaweed is a pure food grown under natural conditions and contains soluble compounds such as nitrates and halogens; chlorides, iodides, bromides, sodium, potassium, calcium, magnesium, aluminium, iron, tin, copper, etc., all of which appear in the human body. Professor G. W. Cavanagh, head of the department of agriculture at Cornell University, says that seaweed contains more than 32 elements, as well as the vitamins A, B, and C. *Dr Weston Price* found while in the Andes that porters carrying heavy loads at between 12-16,000 feet always had little bags of kelp, which they took to strengthen their hearts, and *Dr D. C. Jarvis* prescribed five-grain tablets of kelp after each meal for patients suffering from weak hearts as he found that it banished heart-pain.

Seaweed called 'laver-bread' has always been fried in bacon fat and eaten for breakfast by the Welsh and is one of their national dishes.

Sedatives. Followers of natural therapy do not take sedatives prescribed by orthodox practitioners as they are habit forming and usually have side-effects. For those suffering from stress or sleeplessness there are nervines that will relieve irritation and pain: black haw, bugleweed, mistletoe, skullcap, valerian etc. These may be taken either on their own or in combination with other herbs; in infusions made with boiling water or in pill form. Herbal sedatives are more effective than drugs and can be taken safely.

Seeds. Some kinds of seeds have always been eaten by the human race, usually added to foods to flavour them: poppy and carraway in cakes; cardamom, fenugreek, peppercorns, coriander, cummin, mustard, etc., in curries; fennel was used by the Romans; but till recently seeds were not considered important adjuncts to diet in the West. Indian scientists have discovered recently that during germination peas, cow-peas, mung beans, *rice* and *wheat* contain more *niacin* than when fully mature; the Russians that *soya beans* and *sunflower seeds* are rich in *riboflavin*; and the Hindus and gipsies have always eaten pumpkin seeds for prostate disorders. Sunflower seeds are good for rheumatism and arthritis, and in India sesame seeds are used in the treatment of piles and constipation. Research into seeds continues. Oil is obtained from many of them: peanuts, cottonseed, linseed, sunflower and rape, and more seeds are being grown for their oil, and nutritional and medicinal properties.

Seyle, Dr Hans, MD, Ph.D. An Austrian from a family that has produced four generations of doctors. After earning his MD and Ph.D. from Prague University he studied at Johns Hopkins University, Baltimore and McGill University, Montreal, after which he was appointed head of the University of Montreal's Institute of Experimental Medicine and Surgery.

He had long believed that *stress* was the primary cause of all disease. 'The apparent cause of illness,' he said, 'is often an infection, an intoxication, nervous exhaustion or merely old age. But actually a breakdown of the hormonal-adaption mechanism appears to be the most common ultimate cause of death.' This chemical imbalance of the body he considered was stress. While at McGill he explained his theory to Banting who managed to get him a grant of 500 dollars for experiment, and his results, reported in the *Journal of the AMA* caused a stir throughout the medical world. Today his ideas are accepted and some 5,000 papers are published annually on the subject. His book *Stress,* the first of its kind is a classic which makes sense even to the layman.

Sherman, Henry C. Mitchill Professor of Chemistry at Columbia University, and one of the foremost authorities on food and dietetics. He worked with the US Department of Agriculture, the Food and Nutrition Board of the National Research Council, and the Committee on Nutrition and Food Management of the United Nations Food and Agriculture Association. He enjoys an international reputation and his *Foods: Their Values and Management* is of value to both the scientist and the layman, as are *The Science of Nutrition,* and *Modern Bread From the Viewpoint of Nutrition.* His work on *proteins* has shed a new light on this important food and caused us to change our ideas about it.

Sidhwa, Dr Keki, ND, DO. Born in Bombay, India, on the 29th of September 1926. Graduated at Bombay University and the Edinburgh School of Natural Therapeutics, and later the British School of Naturopathy and Osteopathy. When 14 he was so ill that he was given up by the doctors but his life was saved by a naturopath who put him on a fast. Ever since he has taken a keen interest in natural hygiene and natural living. After graduating from the Kingston Clinic he set up in private practice and founded the Shalimar Health Home at Frinton-on-Sea, Essex. Has travelled extensively in Europe, America and India, talking and lecturing on health. He is the author of a number of books: *Fit For Anything, Problems of Health, Medical Drugs on Trial: Verdict Guilty!* and edits *The Hygienist*. Has written hundreds of articles for health magazines. His three daughters, reared as vegetarians and in the hygienic way of life, have won athletic honours, gold medals in gynmastics, certificates for ballet, and beauty queen contests.

Sidhwa's hobbies are music, philately and long-distance running. To celebrate his 50th birthday he ran 21 miles in three hours; in July 1976 he ran 15 miles in 2 hours 7 minutes in a rain storm to raise money for the American Natural Hygiene Society; and the following month competed in a 10-mile race in Ithica, New York, finishing in 1 hour 22 minutes, coming second in his class – again in pouring rain.

Shalimar is not a fashionable resort where patients are hoodwinked by innumerable gimmicks, but where body, mind and spirit are treated as a whole: by fasting to rid the body of toxins accumulated by faulty living; rest to restore energy and give the organs and tissues a chance to repair themselves; a vegetarian or vegan diet to build up the body; modulated exercises; and postural training in the *Alexander Technique*. Where structural abnormalities exist osteopathic or chiropractic manipulation is given. Finally patients are taught how to eat, live and think before leaving Shalimar.

Sight. See: Eyes.

Silicon. The body of a man weighing 150 lb contains ¼ oz of silicon, a mineral found abundantly in nature in the form of silicon dioxide, or silica in the form of rock crystal, quartz, agate and sand. In the body it prevents disintegration and putrefaction, is a strong antiseptic and a safeguard against epidemic diseases. It is found mainly in hair, nails, feathers and claws in the animal world. In vegetable foods silica is combined with cellulose and forms the skin of fruit and vegetables and the outer coats of cereals, and so is absent in white flour, corn meal, polished rice and processed cereals.

A deficiency of silica lays the body open to many diseased conditions and makes it vulnerable to injury. The hair needs both silica and *sulphur* for growth, so does the enamel of teeth, where it is found in combination with fluorine. Peeling the skins of fruit and vegetables results in a loss of silica, but today when so much food is sprayed they should be scrubbed thoroughly with a stiff brush under flowing water before being eaten.

153

Sinclair, Dr Hugh, MA, DM, B.Sc. One of the leading British Nutritionists; Fellow of Magdalen College, Oxford, and Director of the Laboratory of Human Nutrition, University of Oxford, now in Sutton Courtenay.

Sitz Bath. The sitz bath is an adaptation of the hip bath, having a high sloping back which enables the bather to recline while bathing. The hips, abdomen, bowel region, navel and small of the back are submerged while the chest and lower portions of the thighs are out of water. The sitz bath stimulates and should be taken at temperatures ranging from 74° to 88°F, for from ten to 15 minutes. It is a sovereign treatment for deep-seated digestive and sexual complaints, piles, constipation, sleeplessness and some other disorders. Two or three baths a day should be taken.

For pains, cramp, bowel and bladder troubles, temperatures should range between 100° to 110°F. and the patient should have the upper part of the body wrapped in a blanket and his feet in a rug or muff.

Cold sitz baths, which are invigorating, should be taken in either tepid or cold water – depending on the patient and condition – for from 50 seconds to three minutes, after which the abdomen from the navel down should be rubbed vigorously with a coarse towel; then the patient should be warmed either by a brisk walk or placed in a warmed bed. If properly carried out, sitz baths can be extremely effective.

Skimmed Milk. When milk is allowed to stand the fat globules run together and float to the surface as cream. If the cream is removed the residue is skimmed milk containing from 0.50% to 1.00% fat, depending on the quality of milk. The same result can be achieved more rapidly by a separator in which centrifugal force carries the lighter part of the milk (cream) to the surface, where it is run off. By the separation method less than 0.50% of the fat is retained and the milk is described as 'separated milk'.

Till 1939 skimmed milk was treated as a waste product in Britain and fed to pigs but now we know it to be a valuable food containing all the elements in milk except fat, and dairies have a licence to sell it. Skimmed milk contains *protein* and is rich in calcium. A good deal of skimmed milk is made into low-fat cheese and yogurt. It contains 90.50% water, 3.40% protein, 0.30% fat, 5.10% carbohydrates and 0.70% mineral matter, mainly potassium, calcium and phosphorus, together with the *vitamins A, B* and *D*. It is one of the best foods for the slimmer, being non-fattening and nourishing.

The belief that dried skimmed milk is a poor food is untrue. Unfortunately the product is usually labelled as 'unfit for babies', and as a result is thought to be unfit also for adults. In fact, it is richer in protein, calcium and riboflavin than full-cream milk or skimmed milk.

Skin, The. The skin is not merely a convenient bag that keeps flesh and bones in shape and prevents the blood from escaping. It is the largest organ of the body, containing billions of pores and is connected by the nervous system to every organ and limb. It (1) protects the internal organs from infection and exposure (2) gives the body shape (3) helps to regulate body temperature (4) breathes and absorbs light, air and water (5) exudes poisons through the pores (6) acts as a storehouse for fats and water (7) secretes sebum, a natural lubricant, as well as sweat.

The skin of a man weighing 150 lb harbours about 28 lb of fat and water, and the obese should realise that the skin is a storehouse of excess fat. It reacts to external stimuli and signals pain; if out of condition it becomes hypersensitive, or sensation ceases altogether. When the skin is afflicted by certain diseases such as diabetes, the legs and other portions itch abnormally, as it also does when tight garments such as corsets are worn. When the nerves are destroyed by a disease such as leprosy, the skin can be cut or burned without any sensation of pain. It is tremendously elastic and adjusts itself to loss of weight or the aftermath of pregnancy.

A healthy skin should be free from blemishes such as pimples and boils, which usually indicate that the organs of elimination are not functioning properly or that the wrong foods are being eaten. Psychosomatic conditions also affect the skin, which may break out in a rash when a person is under stress, fear, anxiety or some other severe emotion.

To perspire is an essential function not only for fitness but for existence and the normal adult sweats out about a pint of poisons every 24 hours, leaving a layer of minute waste products on the surface of the skin. If the body is out of condition or the diet faulty this residue will cause an offensive body odour which no amount of perfume or deodorant will mask. Those with offensive body odour should seek the advice of a naturopath or a homeopath, who will provide the appropriate remedies. If the skin is healthy the sweat it gives off will not have an unpleasant odour. During the Vietnam War the Viet Cong said they could smell the body odour of the Americans a long way off and were warned of their presence. The Japanese say that all Westerners have a peculiar body odour.

Heavy meat-eating, and white flour and white sugar products are usually the cause of offensive body odour; or a lack of silica in the system.

After bathing the skin should always be vigorously rubbed with a rough towel to bring the blood to the surface. See: Emotions, Soap.

Sleep. Sleep is essential to health though there are rare instances of people being unable to sleep at all. The normal person, however, would die if kept awake forcibly for more than a week or ten days, and keeping prisoners awake is one form of torture practised in some countries. Sleep rests the body and by some process we do not yet understand, alkalinises the blood. During severe illness the body sometimes loses consciousness, which is nature's way of forcing it to sleep. In most illnesses sound sleep does more to restore the body and pave the way for the recuperating process than pills, potions or tonics. Drugs should not be given during illness when the patient cannot sleep; there are excellent herbs, such as valerian, which achieve the same purpose without having any side-effects.

Slimming. A few people are too fat because they suffer from glandular trouble but most of the obese eat too much, though they do not realise it. Eating is a habit as well as a necessity. If those around you eat, you are tempted to eat as well. The too-fat should ignore the many fancy diets which are sold to the public at inflated prices, and the so-called 'slimming breads', biscuits and made-up foods. The best and wisest way to slim is to eat a little less of everything because the more you eat the greater grows your capacity for food.

No food whatever should be eaten between meals. White sugar and white flour should be eliminated from your diet, and *honey* or *Barbadoes sugar*, and *wholewheat* flour substituted. Gradually the quantities you eat should be decreased till sufficient is consumed to maintain fitness, without a feeling of weakness. Many slimming diets fail because they are too drastic and those who undertake them feel weak and famished and compensate by eating too much. Sudden changes also make many people bad tempered. Most people could live in good health on half the quantity they eat normally.

When your body has accommodated itself to less food you

should try one fast-day a month when you should abstain from all food and take fruit juices only, and then break your fast with fruit and yogurt, followed in the next meal with a salad, eggs, cheese, baked potatoes or nuts. A lacto-*vegetarian* or *vegan* diet is ideal for those who wish to slim; for flesh-eaters fish is best (not herrings) and lean meat. Fasting for more than a day or two should be undertaken only on the advice of a *naturopath*.

The way to know whether you are too fat is to pick up the skin between finger and thumb. If the amount you pick up is more than half an inch thick, then that portion is too fat. A healthy person's ribs can be felt easily and when he inhales they should seen.

Diet should always be accompanied by exercise such as walking, running, skipping, cycling or some other activity that gives pleasure. Games such as tennis, table-tennis, badminton and squash are also effective as they induce sweating, get rid of toxins through the skin, and help to reduce fat.

Under no circumstances should a slimmer resort to drugs, which are habit-forming, or undertake long fasts without proper supervision as these may lead to *anorexia nervosa*, in which one has no desire whatever for food and may have disastrous consequences to health; it may even end in death. See: Diet, Fasting, Vegetarianism, Vegan, Exercise.

Slippery Elm (Red Elm, Moose Elm, and Indian Elm). A native of USA and Canada. The Slippery Elm is a small tree found in profusion in parts of North America. Only the inner bark, which is demulcent, emollient, expectorant, diuretic and nutritive, is used. It is one of the most valuable remedies in herbal medicine for the abundant mucilage it contains, has amazing healing and strengthening properties. It soothes every part in which it comes into contact and may be used either as a gruel to feed infants and sustain invalids, or as a plaster or compress. It forms the basis of many infant-foods. If used as a food it should be mixed into a thin paste and then boiling water should be poured on while it is gently simmered for a minute or two. It may be flavoured with cinnamon, nutmeg, lemon rind and sweetened with honey. Unsweetened, it should be taken for gastritis, mucous colitis and enteritis and is tolerated when no other foods can be retained. It is also of great value in bronchitics, bleeding from the lungs, severe coughs and tuberculosis, and may be used with advantage for other diseases.

The American Indians have for many centuries used the inner

bark to prepare a healing salve. On its own or mixed with marshmallow, it makes the finest poultice known for wounds, boils, ulcers and burns and all inflamed surfaces; soothing, healing and reducing pain and inflammation. There is nothing to touch it for abcesses and boils and gangrenous wounds, either with a mixture of wormwood or very fine charcoal. Slippery elm bark will also preserve fatty substances from becoming rancid; and if a hollow tooth aches and it is not possible to see a dentist, a pinch of slippery elm powder will ease the pain and arrest decay temporarily, though it is in no sense a drug.

Smell, Sense Of. The full enjoyment of food is necessary if it is to produce the maximum benefit. For this a sense of smell as well as *taste* is necessary. Francis Thompson the poet, said that when he was down and out and penniless he would linger on a winter's night on the pavement near the grating above the kitchens of a famous London hotel and savour the odours of the rich foods being prepared, and in this way gained some sustenance even though he never touched a morsel.

Smells are linked with associations and they create *emotions*, good and bad, and we know that emotions can create good health or destroy it. The legendary Dr H. B. Cushing of the Montreal Children's Hospital entered a ward where he was met by Dr R. M. P. Donaghy. 'Have you a case of diphtheria?' he demanded. Donaghy had just meticulously examined a child who had been admitted that morning, then re-examined her before deciding she had diphtheria. 'Why, yes; but how did you know?' he asked.

'I saw an ambulance at the door,' replied Cushing, 'and when I put my head inside the ward I smelled diphtheria.'

Donaghy's diagnosis had taken one hour and 20 minutes; Cushing's four seconds. A good diagnostician can often smell certain diseases on entering a sick room. Wine tasters and perfume experts also have a highly developed sense of smell, and Mr Philip Mayes, lecturer at Leeds University, often uses his sense of smell to detect the sites of kilns when magnetometers have failed. Smell and taste often go together and if one cannot smell a certain dish the taste is usually blotted out or diminished. This was known to mothers in the past, who when giving their children castor oil made them pinch their nostrils together to render the taste less noxious.

The yogis maintained that a person in good health breathes alternately for one hour and 50 minutes through each nostril, a rhythm which is broken during illness, when one nostril usually becomes blocked. During a heavy cold the rhythm can be started again by pressing a small gland under the armpit opposite the blocked nostril. This is in accordance with the theory of *ida* and *pingala* in *yoga* and *yang* and *yin* in *acupucture*. In sleep, though unaware of it, the healthy person turns from one side to the other, to release the flow of air. See: Nose, Taste.

Smoking: See Tobacco.

Sneezing. In sneezing, the abdominal muscles, acting powerfully, push the viscera up against the diaphragm, exerting pressure on the air in the lungs until the tension is sufficient to allow a blast of air to escape by a contraction of the pillars of the fauces and descent of the soft palate, chiefly through the nose, expelling any offending matter present. The famous *William Osler* took snuff once every day in order to sneeze, an exercise, he maintained, that kept him in good health.

Since ancient times, in every part of the world, sneezing has been accompanied by the pious invocation 'God bless you!' or something similar, because the ear and nose were regarded as the gateways to health-giving air *(pneuma)* entering the body and the sneeze was always associated with benefit. The Bible tells us that when Elijah restored the widow's son to life the child sneezed seven times and was well again. George Formby, who made a fortune by singing to the accompaniment of his banjo, was born blind and for three months did not open his eyes. As he was being taken by the Mersey ferry to see a specialist, he sneezed violently – and could see!

Sneezing is not necessarily the sign of a cold coming on; it is well known that printers, who are inveterate snuff-takers, rarely suffer from them.

Soap. The idea that the skin cannot be cleansed without the aid of soap is erroneous. That it is essential has been inplanted in the minds of the public by advertising, put out by soap and detergent manufacturers. Many skin diseases are caused by the *use of too much soap*. Alkalinity of food is desirable, but the skin is not alkaline. It is acid. According to Dr A. L. Hudson, MD, writing in the *Canadian Medical Association Journal* in January 1951, the normal skin has a pH* of from 4 to 6, varying with different parts. Where perspiration is heavy the acidity is greater and during the summer months the pH is even lower. This is the

* Measure of the hydrogen-ion concentration, and hence of the acidity or alkalinity of a solution, expressed on a scale ranging from 0 to 14.

normal condition of healthy skin and is known as the 'acid mantle', which protects the skin from contracting dermatitis and other diseases. When washed with soap, which is alkaline, the 'acid mantle' is destroyed and it may take anything from one to 3½ hours before it recovers normal acidity. During summer the period is less than in winter; that is why many complain of dermatitis or skin irritation in winter, and far fewer in summer.

The acidity of the skin and to some extent its condition depend on the composition of sweat and the amount left unevaporated on the skin. There are conditions other than soap which increase alkalinity of the skin: dust, dirt, disintegrated sweat glands, etc., and skin diseases such as seborrhea, psoriasis get a foothold. Ointments or soaps applied to the body should be acid, not alkaline; once dermatitis has been contracted, alkaline soaps merely exacerbate the condition.

To cleanse the skin it should be washed and rubbed thoroughly with warm water followed (if you can bear it) by cold, and then rubbed vigorously with a rough towel to bring the blood to the surface. For the face (this applies specially to women) warm water and then cold, followed by a cleansing cream, is preferable to soap. Actresses, beauty queens and women who set great store on the condition of the skin on their faces, never use soap – despite what the advertisements say. George Bernard Shaw, who was vain about the condition of the skin on his face, never used soap. Most men, however, shave, and are compelled to use soap, though with the invention of the electric razor their numbers have fallen.

Few can get through the day without collecting grime on their hands: soot, dust, newsprint, etc., and must use soap to get rid of it. The use of soap should be limited to hands, feet, arm-pits and genitals, and a thorough rub over with soap is not necessary more than once a week. The excessive use of soap is responsible for more skin complaints than most people realise.

Ivan T. Sanderson, who spent many years in Africa and wrote knowledgeably on the subject, said that insects attacked only those who used soap, especially house servants and other Africans who had a fetish of washing with soap – a European habit. His wife and other soap-users suffered from bites and those who used soap excessively, from skin infection, but Sanderson and some of the Africans who did not bathe at all were free. What was astonishing is that Sanderson, a scientist, who was constantly hacking himself, falling down and getting abrasions, and handling dead animals, was free from skin infections.

Sodium. A man weighing 150 lb has 2½ oz of sodium in his body. An acid-binding or alkaline element occurs in nature in the form of salts, generally *chloride of sodium* in the sea and in some springs; it also exists as common *salt* in the earth's crust. It has many functions in animal and human organisms: (1) in combination with chlorine it is one of the principal constituents of blood (2) it is necessary for the electric-induction current generated in the nerve spirals by iron in the blood (3) it prevents blood from coagulating too easily (4) plays a part in the formation of saliva, pancreatic juices and bile, and a deficiency of sodium in the blood is one of the principal causes of diabetes because it prevents the system from taking up sufficient oxygen to burn the carbon in food.

Soil. In spite of all that has been written on the subject by recognised authorities the government does not seem to realise that good soil is the basis of health, and if advisers do, then the fertiliser lobby is too powerful for them to persuade farmers to use compost instead of artificials. There is no doubt that food grown in *compost* or *humus* will produce healthy crops immune to disease, and healthier humans who live on them. This has been proved by men like *Sir Albert Howard* and *Sir Jack Drummond*, government advisers on agriculture and food respectively, *Sir Robert McCarrison, Professor Hugh Sinclair, Dr G. T. Wrench, J. I. Rodale, Friend Sykes*, Shewell-Cooper and many others who have devoted their lives to the subject. *The Soil Association*, founded by Lady Eva Balfour, has proved by experiments over a number of years, that crops grown in compost are far more disease-resistant and better for health than those grown in artificials; and Prince Kropotkin, an authority on food, calculated that if all the manure from farm animals was used to make humus, Britain could produce enough food for 100,000,000 people. See: Compost, Humus.

Soil Association, The. Founded by Lady Eva Balfour at New Bells Farm, Haughley, Suffolk, who instigated an experiment by dividing her land into three plots. On one only artificial fertilisers were used; on the second fertilisers and organic materials; on the third only organic materials. On the third plot only compost built up by layers of plant wastes (straw, weeds, etc.), animal manure; soil, chalk and wood ash; and then a final layer of soil, each pile being ventilated by driving a crowbar through the middle or building it round a stake which was subsequently removed.

The Association has proved beyond all question that the third method produces healthy, abundant crops, immune from disease, and if fed to humans and animals, renders them immune as well. See: Compost, Humus.

Sour Milk. Varieties of sour milk have been consumed for centuries throughout the East, North Africa, Greece, Turkey, Russia and Bulgaria but not till comparatively recently in the rest of Europe and America, for in tropical and semi-tropical countries milk curdles easily. Fermented milk drinks such as koumiss and kephir are more easily digested than the milks from which they are made and are often prescribed for patients with chronic catarrh of the stomach or bowels, hepatic cirrhosis and renal disease; sometimes for delirium tremens.

Soya Bean. Of all beans the soya is the most nutritious. The *protein* it contains is as valuable as the casein in milk and it contains all the essential amino-acids, together with *vitamins A*, B_1, B_2, niacin, *vitamin E* and lecithin, and mineral salts. It is an ideal food for vegetarians and vegans. Originally the bean was cultivated in China, Korea and Japan, and in parts of India, and was brought to the notice of the West by the German botanist Englebert Kaempfer at the close of the seventeenth century, but the credit for popularising it must go to the Austrian Fredrich Haberlandt. It is an all-purpose bean and in China an entire banquet made to resemble and tasting of fish, meat, vegetables and sweet, has been made from soya beans alone. It is now widely grown in America, Brazil and parts of Southern Europe.

The bean consists of 10.75% water, 34.00% protein, 16.80% fat, 33.70% carbohydrates and 4.75% minerals, mainly potassium and phosphorus. The bean contains more protein than any other known food but unlike most proteins, is *alkaline*.

Spices. Generally condemned, due to ignorance, by *vegetarians*, *vegans* and *food reformers*, who class them as irritants. And so they are if taken in excess. They are used mainly in pickles and chutnies and in Britain are eaten to give piquancy to tasteless food dished up in cafes and restaurants.

Much store was set on spices in Biblical times, and in the East, Africa and China where the climate can be excessively warm and food putrefies quickly, spices were used in cooking to preserve and impart a distinctive flavour and aroma, for *taste* and *smell* induce digestive juices. Spices are powerful antiseptics and germicides. A *little* added to cooked dishes will improve them; but too much, as of anything, is harmful. Excessively hot curries, chutnies and pickles should be avoided. These are usually eaten by Europeans in the tropics rather than by the natives, who spice their food mildly, enjoy good health and live to a ripe age. If used judiciously, spices improve health.

Coriander, for instance, is an antiseptic and a carminative and in the Middle Ages was one of the ingredients of the renowned Eau de Carmes, made by the Carmelite monks. Cinnamon is a powerful germicide. The scientist Cavel infected beef tea with water taken from a collecting tank in a sewage system and to one sample added cinnamon oil diluted to four parts in 1,000, and to another oil of cloves diluted to two parts in 1,000, and in each sample the germs were destroyed; but carbolic acid to have the same effect had to be used in 5.6 parts in 1,000.

Mace and nutmeg contain volatile oils which are used in renal colic and both aid the digestion and act as a carminative; and *mustard* contains traces of nickel, cobalt and manganese as well as *vitamin D*. Aniseed is eaten to promote appetite and is the basis of innumerable cough mixtures and lozenges. Fennel, saffron and turmeric have health giving properties; cardamom is a digestive, carminative an appetiser; and so is cummin.

The peppers have been valued for centuries for medicinal purposes and in ayurvedic medicine are administered in the form of pills for fevers, for they do not suppress, as does quinine, but cause profuse perspiration, raise the temperature and sweat out poisons. Paprika and the chilli family are rich in vitamin C: Szent Gyorgi isolated a vitamin from paprika juice which is superior to *ascorbic acid* in the prevention of capillary bleeding. He called it *vitamin P* in honour of paprika and permeability.

Ginger and turmeric are used widely in the East for skin diseases, bruises and leech bites.

We are told in Ezekiel 47.12 that the produce of the earth was given to us for sustenance and health: 'and the fruit thereof shall be for meat* and the leaf thereof for medicine.' So use spices in moderation and blend them with foods and they will improve both health and enjoyment.

Spine. Ill treatment of the spine and stomach give rise to most of the diseases with which man is afflicted. We are told, for instance, that back troubles costs the nation more working days

*Food in general; especially solid foods; nuts, vegetables, fruit, eggs, etc. *(OED)*.

each year than industrial disputes. Because millions work in factories stooping over machines or in offices slumped over desks, their spines in due course are thrown out of alignment. The spinal column is a complicated structure consisting of 33 (34 in some people) vertebrae, 23 of which are moveable; 23 cartilages between the vertebrae, and three distinct curves. It isn't straight and a ramrod position is unnatural. The lowest nine or ten vertebrae are partly fused together at the base of the spine into structures known as the *sacrum* and *coccyx* (pronounced kok-ix).

The vertebrae are hollow with the spinal cord passing through them all. Each vertebra is held in place by ligaments, and nerves emerge from the openings between them. Discs between the vertebrae are bound with ligaments which connect bone to bone at each joint and also by muscles running down the length of the spine, and the entire structure is lubricated by *synovial* fluid. Though each vertebra has a very limited movement the sum total of movement of 150 vertebral joints gives the spine astonishing mobility.

If for any reason mechanical strain is imposed on one of these joints it loses much of its normal flexibility, the nerve roots may be pinched and the tissue in the region becomes irritated, swollen and painful.

Each time a movement in any direction is made the muscles of the back are brought into play, but as you grow older – after 40 or 50 – a gradual deterioration sets in and there is a disinclination to bend, especially if you put on weight, and the muscles encasing the spine become stiff and set and ligaments lose their elasticity.

The discs have a soft pulpy interior like marshmallow and if your back is out of condition a sudden jerky movement may tear the casing of a disc so that the pulp protrudes a fraction of an inch and movement of any sort pinches it, causing intense agony. That is why victims of 'slipped discs' become fixed.

The cure lies not in the hands of the orthodox physician, who will usually place the patient in a plastic collar or rigid waistcoat, preventing further movement, and sometimes making a surgical operation necessary. An osteopath or chiropractor should be consulted, who will apply pressure in the right places, or manipulate the back, breaking down lesions so that the disc will slip into place, relieving pain. Then he may further manipulate and advise remedial exercises for it is lack of exercise together with the wrong sort of food that brings about this painful condition.

The spine needs constant exercise if it is to remain in good condition throughout a long life.

Spirits. If you have not already started drinking – don't. That is the safest rule. Whereas brandy, whisky and rum have no food value whatever, thay have their uses. Charles Robb, Professor of Surgery at London University, said: 'I think the best thing for the relief of pain is alcohol. I don't mean anything pharmaceutical – but whisky. We put our patients on big and repeated doses of whisky up to the maximum tolerance in individual cases. But this, of course, is a short term method and should not be used for chronic cases.' In certain diseases alcohol is given as it dilates blood vessels and aids circulation and is better than drugs.

The French call brandy *eau de vie,* literally 'water of life,' for it has kept alive many a patient with fluttering heart or angina at a critical moment. Dr A. Lapthorne Smith said that when he was 45 a relative was given a hogshead (100-140 gallons) of very old Jamaica rum by the husband of a lady whose life he had saved. This rum he bequeathed to Dr Lapthorne Smith who each night took two ounces of the spirit in hot water with two lumps of sugar. When he was 90 he still had a few bottles left. He drank no other liquor and ate wisely and in moderation. If spirits are indulged in in such moderation they will do no harm. Unfortunately they seldom are. See: Alcohol, Beer, Wine.

Sprouting Beans. The first record we have of sprouting beans being eaten is in China in 2838 BC. The soya, the mung and in fact, all beans can be sprouted to produce an especially valuable vegetable in mid-winter when fresh vegetables are scarce. Mung beans are a good source of *vitamins A* and *B* and are very rich in C. Soya beans contain an enzyme which tends to oxidise and destroy ascorbic acid (vitamin C) when the sprouts are chopped and exposed to the air, but if boiled for two minutes the enzyme is destroyed and none of the vitamin lost.

When the beans are soaked for four hours some vitamin C is formed, equal to that in tomato juice, but after storage in a refrigerator for seven days the amount doubles, after which it deteriorates.

For sprouting, use only clean whole beans. Wash and place them in a large shallow dish and cover with roughly four times their volume of lukewarm water. The beans will swell to six times their original volume. Soak overnight – no longer – then drain off water, rinse and drain again. Cover with a cheesecloth or fine mesh screen; tie securely, invert the dish on to a pan and place in a warm spot at a slightly tilted angle. Place the dish under a flowing tap of cold water three times a day to wash away mould or bacteria, then return to inverted position. In three or four days at room temperature (70°F) the sprouts should be from one to two inches long and ready for use. See: Wheat.

Still, Dr Andrew Taylor. Born in Virginia, USA, in 1828 of a Scots mother and English-German father. Served as a surgeon in the Union Army during the Civil War. One day while hiding in the woods in Kansas a fellow officer, Major Abbot, confided: 'Do you know, I have lost all faith in Medicine? I am satisfied that it is all wrong and that the system of drugs as curative agents will one day be practically overturned and some other system or method of curing the sick will take its place.' After the war Still felt that he was destined to be that agent.

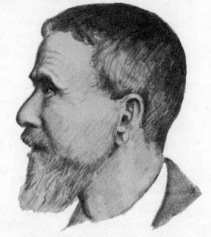

He had always been a student of Nature and insisted that the body was a perfect machine which will function smoothly if allowed

Dr Andrew Taylor Still

to do so. He said: 'The rule of the artery must be absolute, universal and unobstructed, or disease will be the result'. It is on this principle that osteopathy was founded. He maintained that all diseases are mere effects and the causes must be found in order to restore health. As the relations of the tissues of the body are determined by their relations to the bony framework, he turned his attention to the skeleton and for years wandered the country as a bonesetter, eventually setting up in practice in Kirksville, Missouri. In 1887 he started to teach his four sons the art and in 1892 founded the American School of Osteopathy, a word derived from the Greek *osteon*, bone, and *pathos*, feeling. He engaged Dr William Smith, a graduate from Edinburgh, to teach Anatomy and Physiology, and after a period conferred the first diploma in Osteopathy on him. In 1894 the training, which took two years and was occupied mainly with the study of

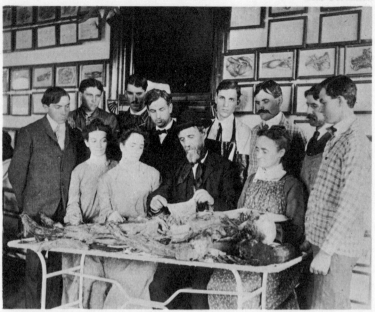

Dr Andrew Still, founder of Osteopathy instructing students round a dissecting table at the turn of the century

Anatomy and Osteopathy, was extended till today osteopaths undergo a course comparable with that of the orthodox medical student.

In 1902 Dr Willard Walker and Dr F. J. Horn were encouraged by a wealthy Bostonian to emigrate to London and set up in osteopathic practice, and a few months later Dr Jay Dunham and Dr Harvey Foote were sent to Belfast by an Irish-American millionaire to treat his paralysed sister, who was cured and sent to America. All four doctors remained and the osteopathic invasion of Britain had begun. See: Osteopathy.

The Stomach. Dr Samuel Johnson, who used to pontificate on every subject under the sun, once made this very sound observation: 'He who will not mind his belly will hardly mind anything else.'

The stomach, a vital organ, is protected by layers of muscle which can be strengthened and toughened by exercise. These consist of: (1) a layer of translucent membrane – serous coat (2) a coat of involuntary muscle in three layers – muscular coat (3) a layer of connective tissue containing blood vessels – submucous

167

coat (4) a ring of muscle – pylorus. To look at some men's stomachs you would think they had only one coat and that composed entirely of blubber.

A fat stomach is an invitation to hernia, constipation and a host of related diseases. Dr William Parsons of Virginia University, said that fat people are more likely to contract heart disease, diabetes, liver diseases and gall-stones than those of normal weight; and Dr J. H. Tilden that 'Fat people excrete into their own bodies', a most unpleasant thought. A fit person has a fit stomach.

Stress. In a Report to the Congress of Mental Health in London in 1968 Dr Jonathan Gould said that at least ten per cent of children in Britain under the age of 15 were exposed to stress which eventually will affect their mental development. Dr W. M. S. Russell says that crime rates have risen because of stress, and Dr E. E. Lieber stated in the journal *Personnel Management* that neurosis caused by stress, resulted in a loss to industry of nearly 20,000,000 man-hours each year. This was endorsed by the Office of Health Economics, which disclosed that 32,000,000 working days were lost through mental illness in 1966 at a cost to the NHS of £140,000,000. Lord Balniel, Chairman of the National Association for Mental Health estimates that one out of every nine girls now aged six will enter a mental home at some period of her life and Lord Taylor, a distinguished physician, that one in three Britons suffers from 'a sub-clinical neurosis syndrome.' Nor are students immune from stress for a survey in 1963 revealed that one in seven of the 100,000 university students in Britain needs mental treatment, and Nottingham University had appointed a full-time psychiatrist. Because stress cannot be diagnosed with the same certainty as organic diseases it is the greatest menace in our society. See: Emotions, Seyle.

Sugar. The idea that refined (white) sugar is a food is false. It has a high calorific value and the most it can do is to provide instant energy. There are other edibles, however, which have food value and provide instant energy as well: *honey, molasses* and dried fruit. White sugar is a slow poison and an irritant and taken daily over a long period lays the foundation to many diseases, the most common of which are diabetes, dental caries, impaired sight, arteriosclerosis and coronary thrombosis. Professor John Yudkin, Emeritus Professor of London University, said; 'High sugar content in diet causes figures for coronary thrombosis to be at least five times as high or more, so that translating this you would see that if people stopped eating sugar you could reckon on saving 80,000 to 100,000 lives in Great Britain alone.

'Taking the other related diseases such as arteriosclerosis into account, the number of lives you could save by stopping people from eating sugar could be from 250,000 to 300,000.'

Refined sugar contains no vitamins and is devoid of mineral salts, and *saccharine* and cyclamates are even more harmful and have been condemned by the FDA* in America. Pure cane juice, raw sugar, molasses and black treacle contain significant quantities of mineral matter, but the amounts in white sugar, Demerara, barley sugar, caramel and golden syrup are negligible. Taken over a long period these lead to degenerative diseases. Unfortunately, the British are the biggest consumers of sugar and tins of fruit and jam from Australia and South Africa contain more sugar than those meant for other markets. Sugar accounts mainly for the nation's bad teeth. Dr Carlton Fredericks says that all forms of sugar are toxic and the leading medical authorities and dieticians in Germany, France, America and Britain agree with him. See: Glucose, Saccharin, Honey.

Sulphur. The body of a man weighing 150 lb contains 3½ oz of sulphur, which is found in the elementary state mixed with earthy material in volcanic regions, chiefly in Sicily, Nevada and California. It is a yellow, brittle, solid substance with neither taste nor odour, is insoluble in water and melts at 239°F. Sulphur is chiefly taken up by the animal organism in the form of protein and is a constituent of the haemoglobin of blood, where it serves as an oxidising agent. It enters into the composition of albumen, gelatin, etc., in the tissues. It is one of the elements which give the body its power of resistance to disease, as the organising sulphuric acid salts have a cleansing and antiseptic influence in the alimentary canal. Sulphur should be taken in organic form in fruits and vegetables but not in any quantity through mineral waters. It is carried in the stems and leaves of plants, the skins of fruit, and in seeds.

Sultanas. A species of dried grape, which like raisins and currants are rich in fruit sugar and a good source of energy. They contain virtually the same properties. See: Raisins, Currants.

Sunflower Seeds. As long ago as 1901 *Dr Harvey W. Wiley,* head of the Department of Agriculture, USA, stated in Bulletin N 60 that there existed an old-folks' tale that eating sunflower seeds cured

*Food and Drug Administration.

rheumatism, and it was found that at state banquets in China the seeds were always placed in bowls on the table and munched between courses. *J. I. Rodale* found evidence that the seeds not only cured rheumatism but many cases of arthritis as well, and in some instances improved eyesight. Members of the Lewis and Clark Expedition to Montana in 1805 placed it on record that the Indians, who enjoyed remarkable health and stamina used the seeds as food, hair oil and soap, and flour made from them for bread and thickening soups. The sunflower is easy to grow and every gardener should put down a row. There are many varieties, which grow from four to 30 feet but the average, which produces a good flower reaches eight feet and has a diameter of 24 inches. The finest sunflowers are to be found in tropical and semi-tropical countries, but they grow well in British soil.

The seeds have an astonishing effect on the nervous system. When in 1974 Clare Nessholme aged seven, daughter of a biochemist at Oxford University became paralysed by polyneuritis (Guillain-Barre syndrome) and doctors gave up all hope of a recovery, her parents after studying scientific literature, gave her one teaspoon of sunflower oil a day and restricted animal fats. Her condition improved almost immediately. Some months later she was able to hold her right hand almost vertically for ten seconds; after two months she could feed herself; the following month she walked six paces unaided, and the following year she enrolled in a ballet class! One case does not constitute proof but there are many instances of sunflower seeds helping victims of multiple sclerosis. The seeds are exceptionally rich in *thiamin, niacin, vitamins D, E, F* and *K* and linoleic acid. Dr H. T. Slover of the Human Nutrition Research Division, USA, found that the seeds contain four times as much vitamin E as corn and soya beans. Analysis reveals: 7.50% water, 14.20% protein, 32.30% fat, 14.50% carbohydrates and 3.50% mineral matter, mainly calcium and phosphorus.

Sun Bathing. A popular and healthful pastime in temperate countries and almost a mania in Sweden, Norway, Finland and other regions where the winter is long and dark and there is a scarcity of sun.

Sunlight has a beneficial effect on the human body but too much can be harmful. From ancient times men have worshipped the sun: the Incas and Aztecs had sun gods; Zoroastrians turn towards the sun when they worship; yogis perform their *surya namaskars* (salutation to the sun) while facing it. *Finsen, Rollier,* Gauvain and others made the world aware of the curative power of sunlight in the treatment of tuberculosis, rickets and skin diseases, for sunlight has the power to kill certain kinds of bacteria, and when the sun's rays fall on the skin the ultraviolet rays activate a pro-vitamin which already exists in it and vitamin D is formed in the body.

Sunlight aids and stimulates the healing of wounds and has cured cases of asthma and hay fever, though it has made some cases worse. No one knows why. It improves appetite and nutrition and the capacity to assimilate and metabolise food; creates a sense of well-being and an increase in muscular strength; benefits the glands, the lymphatic vessels and tissue; increases lung capacity; stimulates the action of the heart and circulation and, if the blood pressure is not too high, the ultraviolet rays acting on the skin and indirectly on the pancreas, tend to lower blood pressure. If the blood pressure is too low the sun's rays stimulate the adrenal glands and raise it to normal.

Sunshine increases the number of blood cells and the colouring matter in blood; it increases also the number of phagocytes, which help to resist harmful bacteria; increases the oxidising capacity of blood and lowers its sugar content and so is a valuable aid in the fight against diabetes. Sunshine eliminates poisons from the system, brings relief to victims of gout, rheumatism and lumbago, conditions produced by toxins and acids; stimulates the nervous system, makes hypochondriacs forget their symptoms and generally has a stimulating effect. In countries with too little sun it helps to cure anaemia, insomnia and irritability.

Unless foods containing calcium and phosphorus are eaten, however, the body will not release the *vitamin D* which is activated by the sun's rays; and much of the beneficial ultra-violet rays will be lost if one sits behind glass, even special vita-glass through which only a percentage of the rays can pass.

Sunshine should be imbibed in small doses at first; at mid-day for not more than five minutes at a stretch until the skin gradually browns, when a layer of dark pigment under the skin traps the rays and renders them harmless. People with dark skins can absorb far more sun without burning than those with fair skins, and for the red-haired the sun can be poison for ginger folk burn easily unless they inure themselves gradually to its rays. In America in 1976 more than 12,000 sunbathers were admitted

171

into hospital – many with severe eye damage – mostly women under 25 who had fallen asleep under sun lamps.

Sunshine is a mixed blessing. Never roast in the sun for according to Dr W. Hunter, Medical Officer of West Bridgeforth: 'Long exposure of the body is positively harmful. It may be dangerous by causing skin irritation, which may eventually lead to a pre-cancerous condition and actual cancer on the exposed parts of the body.' Switzerland, where the sun is worshipped, has the highest cancer mortality in the world.

When sun-bathing, don't use sun tan lotions with a lanoline base as these can cause *allergy*; avoid drugs and alcohol – even aspirins – and take your sunshine in small doses interspersed with dips in the sea or river.

Sweating. For perfect health one should sweat profusely once a day for the pores are the channel through which the body gets rid of some of its wastes. When the Ancient Greeks who were noted for their physical prowess exercised, they first rubbed themselves with olive oil, then dusted their bodies with fine powder to close the pores and prevent excessive perspiration, which kept the body cool and free from chills. After vigorous exercise, oil, powder and sweat were scraped off with an instrument called a strigil and the body was bathed. Professor J. Strasburger, who wrote the section on Hydrotherapy in Krause's *Lehrbuch*, said: 'The overheating of the body and perspiration aid one to perfection, and in the combination of overheating and perspiration is to be found the reason why sweating is curative in rheumatic diseases of the muscles and in many other diseases. By means of experiments it has been shown that sweat is poisonous; perspiration contains not only poisons in solution, but certain gases. The perspiration of different races and different individuals smells differently. It is not sufficiently clear how far bacterial poisons consequent upon infection can be eliminated in perspiration but it has been asserted that the sweating of the tuberculous is a method of Nature of eliminating tubercular poisons. At any rate sweating is a natural method of ridding the surface of the body, and particularly the creases of the skin and its openings, from dirt and bacteria. Thus disinfection of the skin is effected.' See: Skin, Soap.

Sykes, Friend. Sykes started farming with Friesian cattle and Berkshire pigs in 1916 and by 1923 his cattle and pigs were ranked among the best in Britain, winning innumerable awards and trophies. Encouraged by his success he turned to the breeding of thoroughbreds, again with equal success. But the finest horses can be raised only on the right kinds of grasses, clovers and herbs and on land with a subsoil of either limestone or chalk. So he sold out and moved to Chute in Wiltshire, to a high lying farm with poor topsoil, on Salisbury Plain. By using a subsoiler before ploughing and treating the surface with humus made from straw, farm wastes, weeds and similar refuse he rejuvenated the land and made his farm into one of the most fertile in the country, on which animals free from, and resistant to, disease were raised, for he was a disciple of *Albert Howard*. He studied the land, kept records and wrote books, among which *Humus and The Farmer*, a classic of its kind, shows how any farmer can achieve similar results.

He believed that Man is the product of the food he eats, which applies equally to animals, and when some of his mares failed to foal he added wheat germ to their fodder, with astonishing results. He condemned the practice of cutting down hedges to give more space for crops and planted trees and coppices where birds and small animals could drink and take refuge, for they added to the farmer's prosperity and enriched the land. He believed that worms were the farmer's greatest friend and did all he could to encourage them, as he did weeds. Artificial fertilizers, insecticides and poisonous sprays were never used on his fields. He was a conservationist long before conservationism became popular and, working with Nature, he reaped ample rewards. He foretold of a 'Black Death', which we can see looming ahead, and predicted that dust bowls would render large tracts of America and Canada into deserts because bad farming had eroded the topsoil and high winds would blow it away – which is what happened. See: Compost, Humus, Soil.

Synthetic Vitamins. There are authorities – usually men with degrees in chemistry – who assure us that vitamins manufactured in the laboratory from chemicals are every bit as good as those which Nature had placed in fruit, vegetables, roots, flowers and weeds; that white bread from which the bran, outer coats of the grain and wheat germ have been removed, and synthetic vitamins substituted, is every bit as good as wholewheat. Either such people know little about food in relation to health, or have a commercial interest in producing synthetic vitamins or processed foods.

Vitamin C, which consists of six parts of carbon, eight of hydrogen and six of oxygen can be extracted from citrus fruit, tomatoes, paprika, etc., but it can also be made far more cheaply from coal tar chemicals and 99% of the vitamin C now sold is from this source. But the vitamin made synthetically is never as effective as that extracted from natural sources. There is no doubt that natural vitamins far exceed in health-giving properties and potency those produced from chemicals. Isobel W. Jennings of Cambridge University pointed out in *Vitamins in Endocrine Metabolism* that whereas synthetic vitamins perform some of the functions of their natural counterparts they are ineffective in others, even though their chemical structure is identical. She added that excessive doses of natural vitamins are harmless as they are generously diluted in plant and animal substances; but they are usually toxic in their synthetic state if very large doses are taken.

Dr. S. Ayres, Jr, MD, stated in the *Journal of The American Medical Association* that in the case of vitamin E, though chemically identical, the natural and synthetic forms polarized light differently, the natural vitamin being far more active. This was borne out by Drs Evan V. Shute and William Shute, pioneers in the field of vitamin E therapy.

Dr William Ellis and colleagues of The Natural Food Associates, stated that natural vitamin C contains micronutrients lacking in the synthetic product, and Dr R. Peterman, MD, stated in the *JAMA** that vitamin A, as it occurs naturally in food presents no problems, no matter how much we take; but this is not so in the case of synthetic vitamin A.

The Russians carried out experiments with vitamin C in 1946, reporting the results in *Vitamin Research News*, No. 1, 40. They fed a number of mice on a deficient diet causing them all to contract scurvy, then divided them into two groups. The first, fed on natural vitamin C, recovered rapidly and were all cured; the other, given synthetic C, responded slowly, and some even failed to respond, and died.

In *Food and Nutrition* E. W. H. Cruikshank, MD, described an experiment in which chicks were fed on the same diet and then divided into three groups. One received no vitamin D at all; the second was given synthetic D; and the third natural D. In the no-vitamin group 60 chicks died; those fed on synthetic D gained 346 grammes in weight; and those given natural D, 399 grammes.

Nutrition Review Vol. 5, pp 251-253, 1947, published an article

*Journal of The American Medical Association

on *The Relative Activity of Natural and Synthetic Vitamin E* in which it was shown that the natural vitamin was three times as potent as synthetic vitamin E.

Sister Justa Smith, Ph.D, a Franciscan nun who is Assistant Director of Education at Rosewall Park Memorial Institute for Cancer Research in Buffalo, New York, and Director of Research for the Human Dimensions Institute, has carried out hundreds of experiments on tissues and organs to find out why healing takes place. She believes that every cell in the body has its nutritional needs, which during illness must be deficient in one or more of these. So she decided to test natural and synthetic vitamins by means of a technique known as paper chromatography in which the substance tested leaves distinctly coloured shapes on filter paper. The synthetic vitamin C left a pattern of concentric circles; the natural vitamin C produced rays from the centre and a fluted perimeter, proving that the natural vitamin was different and probably possessed some substance lacking in the synthetic one.

Semyon and Valentina Kirlian, Russian scientists, who are pioneers in a form of photography by which the auras of plants and leaves can be detected, have shown that natural vitamins throw off a luminosity not seen in synthetic products.

This does not mean that synthetic vitamins have no value. They have, but where there is a choice always take natural vitamins instead of synthetic, and preferably get your vitamins from fruit and vegetables grown in *compost* rather than pills and capsules.

See: Vitamins.

Szent-Györgyi, A. A Hungarian scientist who in 1928 recovered a crystalline substance from the adrenal cortex, oranges and cabbages which proved to be anti-scorbutic. He and Svirvely, a colleague, gave it to guinea-pigs suffering from scurvy and cured them. He also discovered a rich source of this substance in paprika and sent a sample to the laboratory at Birmingham University where its structural formula was worked out and the compound synthesized. It was found that the substance could take up oxygen and also be reduced and that doses of 30 milligrammes a day prevented scurvy. 'The more I learnt about this substance,' wrote Györgyi, 'the more interesting it seemed to be. Eventually I crystallised it. It was an acid and seemed related to an unknown sugar which I called "ignose," so the substance itself was called "ignostic acid." But the Editor of the journal to which I sent my paper did not like jokes and rejected the name. 'Godnose' being no more successful, we agreed that the child's name should be 'hexuronic acid.' Later, with the advancing knowledge of its structure it had to be rebaptised and is now called ascorbic acid because it is identical with vitamin C and prevents scurvy. In this way I became the father of a vitamin.' In plant tissues there is an oxidase which, when the cell is damaged, destroys the ascorbic acid and this has a bearing on the marketing, cooking and preparation of fruits and vegetables for the table. In order to retain the ascorbic acid there should be the minimum of cutting, chopping and bruising.

T

Taste. Though not an infallible guide, taste plays an important part in health. Food you enjoy often does more good than that which you dislike but which is supposed to be beneficial. Tastes differ widely with individuals though the four varieties of taste – sweet, sour, salt and bitter – can be blended in foods to suit all palates. As in the case of colours, one taste can give a person pleasure but nauseate or repel another. Taste is often associated with colour and purple, grey, and black are the least popular colours for foods.

Many tastes are either acquired or hereditary though in some instances a desire for certain substances is dictated by elements your body may lack. Pregnant women, for instance, often hanker for foods they normally would not think of eating; and tastes can change during disease such as pernicious anaemia, diabetes, diseases of the pharynx and cancerous growths on the tongue. Dr Kathleen Vaughan says that in Kashmir there were three indigenous cures for 'trouble in the bones': (1) a special clay called Baramulla earth (2) pills made from fish liver (3) rubbing wounds with mustard oil and exposing them to *sunlight*. A lump of Baramulla earth taken from a patient suffering from osteomalacia, who ate pieces of it, was analysed by the Clinical Research Association and found to contain 16.20% of calcium phosphate, 11.80% of ferric oxide, 71.20% of hydrated aluminium silicate and 0.80% of undetermined residue. Patients ate this earth instinctively.

In 1961 the first case of cobalt deficiency was recorded in Monmouthshire when a 16-month-old child crawled around and swallowed earth from flower pots. The soil in which her food was grown was found to be lacking in cobalt and when she was treated with cobaltous chloride flavoured with blackcurrant syrup she ceased to hanker after earth, slept well and started to look vital and intelligent.

Loss of ability to taste is sometimes caused by injections of D-penicillamine or by a deficiency of niacin or *riboflavin in* the system.

Tears. Tears are the expression of grief peculiar to the human race in the animal kingdom. They act like steam in a boiler which when the pressure rises too high is ejected through the safety valve. If tears do not flow during extreme grief something in the system may break down. Tears relieve tension. Women are biologically stronger than men and live longer, partly because they cry more easily. Dr Erich Lindemann said that bereaved patients unable to weep invariably complained of depressing symptoms. He discovered during one period that 33 out of 41 patients with ulcerative colitis developed their disease because of pent-up emotions. In 1967 Dr David Kissen told the International Conference on Chest and Heart Diseases in Glasgow that people with poor emotional outlets had almost four and a half times the risk of developing lung cancer than normal people. Crying is a nervously controlled and directed act which involves the central nervous system and the obstruction of tears instinctively results in tensions.

Incidentally, tears contain lysozme, one of Nature's finest antiseptics, which in the process of being released kills bacteria. Weeping for joy also serves the same purpose as weeping for grief, as it releases pent-up emotions, and women who go to the cinema and 'weep buckets' during romantic films are, unwittingly, doing themselves much good.

Men should not be ashamed to weep when overcome by intense grief, such as caused by the death of a near relative, or when overcome by intense emotion. Indiscriminate weeping by women who 'turn on the tap' when frustrated or because they want something badly, is, of course, to be deplored. It then becomes a weapon. Such weeping is a form of blackmail. See: Emotions.

Teeth. Teeth are an integral part of the human body and not pieces of bone placed in the gums independent of the remainder. They depend for their health on nourishment just as organs and limbs do. Each tooth consists of: (1) a crown which projects beyond the level of the gum (2) neck, which is just below the crown (3) root, which is embedded in the gum. The top layer consists of hard material called dentine or ivory, below which is the pulp consisting of loose connecting tissue, blood vessels and nerves, and under the dentine is a layer of cement. Nerves enter the tooth from openings at the extreme end of the root. When decay sets in the enamel erodes, the nerve is exposed, and toothache is the result. Toothache is Nature's warning that action should be taken to cover the nerve, which is done by drilling a cavity and filling it with a hard substance.

Toothache will recur if decay in the cavity is not removed. When the dentist's ministrations are complete, however, decay can be prevented only by eating the right sort of food: raw fruit, vegetables in the form of salads, nuts and milk products, and eggs and fish such as herrings and halibut. In this way the teeth will be supplied by the *vitamins A, D and C;* calcium and phosphorus. A raw carrot or nuts after each meal will clean the surfaces of the teeth and prevent food from adhering to them, which is one cause of caries. White flour products and sugar should be banished from the diet.

Chewing raw fruit and nuts and other hard substances, exercises the gums, though nuts should not be cracked by the teeth as the shells are harder than enamel and likely to chip it. Chewing does not harm the teeth. Eskimos eat such tough food that their teeth are often worn to half their size, yet they never suffered with toothache till they were introduced to a civilised diet. Mastication assists the production of saliva, aids the process of digestion, and people who lose all their teeth and suffer from indigestion would be well advised to have themselves fitted with dentures. See: Fletcherism.

Temperance. This is the habit or practice of restraining oneself from excessive eating, drinking and other desires. It is now applied erroneously to teetotalism. The sensible person is temperate in all things and the better for it. See: Alcohol, Beer, Wine, Spirits.

Temperature of The Body. Though it is generally accepted that normal body temperature should be 98.4 degrees F., temperature differs in people from 35.5C to 37.5C (97.0F to 99.0F). It depends on the difference of heat produced and heat lost and vigorous muscular exercise may raise it by one degree Centrigrade. If in normal health the temperature rarely stays either above or below normal for more than a few minutes. Alcohol in large doses is one of the poisons that upsets the body's thermostat; that is why drunks often die from over-exposure in winter. Whisky, brandy, gin, rum and vodka raise the temperature only temporarily.

A rise in temperature is Nature's warning that the system has been upset in some way; some tissue or organ has been damaged and, says Dr David Gocke, professor of Medicine at Columbia University, 'the body responds with an inflammatory reaction. In infection, for instance, the body tries to get rid of damaged tissue. White blood cells (leucoytes) infiltrate the area and devour the damaged tissue so that it can be carried off. In the process the white cells themselves break down and die, releasing pyrogens (heat-producing substances) which circulate in the brain and there prod the thermostat into action. Body temperature rises and fever results.'

Shivering and fever generate internal heat, boost the temperature higher, causing loss of appetite, nausea and weakness, and sometimes a stomach upset. As the temperature soars the body's thermostat issues emergency signals to the vital organs and in the fight to cool your blood, vessels in your skin dilate, your face flushes, your heart beats faster, blood flows more rapidly to flush out damaged cells, making room for new healthy ones. Eventually, when your inside is warm again the warmth reaches the skin; you sweat and the cooling process lowers your temperature.

When you have a high temperature (about one or two degrees above normal) you should go straight into a warm bed, refuse all food for at least 24 hours (preferably 48) and drink a hot infusion of elderflower, yarrow and peppermint (or capsicum) which will make you sweat profusely and help to get rid of some of the wastes inside you. If you don't have such herbs in the house, plenty of warm water with or without lemon juice will serve, and there is no reason why a stiff tot of brandy, whisky or rum should not be added. At the end of 24 hours you should feel much better. No nostrum any NHS doctor can prescribe is half as good as a warm bed, complete rest and a fast. All you can do is assist Nature, and the hot drinks do just that. Never try to suppress a temperature, as it is part of the healing process. See: Fasting, Herbs.

Thompson, Kenneth and Angela. Run *yoga* classes at Brentwood Evening Institute and Redbridge Social Centre, where students are given remedial exercise, taught *food reform* and how to care

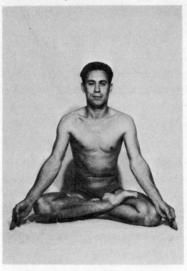

Ken Thompson in the Lotus pose

for their health. Thompson, who started the venture, was small and puny but like so many of his kind wanted to be strong and healthy, so embraced *yoga* which brought him unusual health and strength and gave him the energy to play badminton, tennis and soccer with unusual skill, and take up weight-training and gymnastics. His wife became a yoga disciple and they aim at developing physique and widening the spiritual development of their pupils. He and his wife have brought health to hundreds.

Thomson, James C. (1887-1960). Founder of the Kingston Clinic, Edinburgh, and famous as the main protagonist, with *Stanley Lief,* of the Nature Cure Home in Britain. Son of a farmer born in the county of Angus, and a relative of David Livingstone and J C. Thomson, inventor of the pneumatic tyre.

At 16 he became a lawyer's assistant but joined the Royal Navy and within two years went down with a lung infection. He was discharged and sent home as the surgeon said he had no more than three months to live; but Thomson decided to fight for his life. Before enlisting he had made friends with a number of students at the Edinburgh Medical School, one of whom was an advocate of *hydrotherapy*, physical culture and *diet reform*. Thomson, in desperation, bought books on these subjects, devoured them and set out to cure himself. He went to a Perthshire farm belonging to a cousin and every day prayed that the bleeding from his lungs would stop. One day he suddenly realised it had – and the haemorrhage stopped for a week! He rapidly regained health, developed his body and joined the Metropolitan Police but when offered promotion to the CID resigned and emigrated to America.

His first call was to *Macfadden* and then to Dr Henry Lindlhar at his Sanitarium in Chicago, where he became a pupil: He was so keen and tireless that within a comparatively short time he was made Manager. Wrestling, weight-lifting and long-distance walking transformed him into a powerful man. He specialised in studies of the mind and was trained to handle mentally deranged patients.

He wanted his own practice, however, so despite offers of much more money went to Missouri where he set up a flourishing health home and was known as 'The Sunshine Doctor'. From there he moved to Florida where a wealthy patient asked him to become her personal physician and offered him half a mile of beach as a gift. Had he accepted, that strip would have brought him more than a million dollars when Miami was turned into a pleasure resort for the rich, but the climate did not suit him and he hankered after the bracing air of Edinburgh. There during the First World War he started a naturopathic practice and after many vicissitudes and an extended tour of the United States, established a clinic in the heart of the capital's medical world, with a nursing home on one side of him and the BMA offices on the other. He also ran a free clinic for the prevention and correction of deformities in children whose parents were too poor to pay.

He lectured, wrote books and pamphlets, started a magazine and with the help of his wife and sisters made a resounding success of the venture and eventually opened the famous Kingston Clinic a few miles outside Edinburgh. The medical and legal authorities harrassed and persecuted him and did their utmost to destroy his practice; he was even falsely accused of speeding and given a jail sentence; but he fought these prosecutions, emerged with credit and made the Kingston Clinic, where more than 75,000 people from all over the world have been treated, famous. Today certificates for sickness benefit issued by the Clinic have been officially recognised and the success of the Clinic has been testified to in Parliament (*Hansard* 18.2.1946).

Tissue Salts. See: Scheussler, Biochemic remedies.

Tobacco. Smoking is a social habit indulged in universally and, like all habits, does no harm in strict moderation. But it can undermine the system and athletes, for instance, should not smoke if they want to give of their best. Smoking can be a tranquilliser and in these times when *stress* affects so many millions, soothes the nerves of those who smoke. Smoking is far preferable to the use of drugs for settling the nerves.

Pipes and cigars are preferable to cigarettes but even heavy pipe smokers have gone completely blind because the optic

181

nerve has been destroyed by toxic deposits. No one who suffers in any way from eye trouble should smoke; nor should sufferers from bronchitis, asthma, and tuberculosis. Burger's disease, which for some unknown reason is prevalent among Jewish people, occurs in 50% of heavy smokers; and it also leads to sclerosis of the arteries and to subsequent gangrene. Smoking is a senseless costly habit but telling people not to smoke will not prevent millions from adopting the habit; if you don't smoke however, don't start. If you do, limit yourself to five filter-tipped cigarettes a day, or to two small cigars or two pipes a day. And – do not inhale.

Tomato. A native of tropical America; the name comes from the Spanish *tomate*. It was eaten raw and used in cooking by the Mexicans and Indians before them. In Europe it was originally called the love-apple and was supposed to possess aphrodisiac properties. Though used mainly as a vegetable in Britain it is a species of berry and belongs to the family *Solanacae*. Once it was thought to be poisonous. The sweetest tomatoes and those richest in *vitamin C* are grown in tropical and semi-tropical countries, for they thrive in the sun. They were at first regarded with suspicion by Europeans until in 1793 they were accepted as a vegetable in the markets of Marseilles. The tomato can be eaten raw or cooked; made into jams, chutnies and pickles; or as is often done in the tropics, sliced, sprinkled with sugar or mixed with honey, topped with cream or yogurt and eaten as a sweet. It consists of 94.00% water, 0.90% protein, 0.20% fat, 3.75% carbohydrates and 1.28% mineral matter, mainly potassium, phosphorus, calcium and sulphur. In addition to vitamin C, the tomato contains A and K.

Tongue. Organ of speech and taste and an indicator of disease. An old medical saying is that a red tongue needs alkaline and a white tongue acids; blueness that the blood is not getting enough oxygen; and a dry tongue denotes a poor appetite. Dyspepsia is shown by a large, pale, flabby tongue. If pressed by the teeth it remains indented. Disease is also indicated by the tongue. Diabetes is accompanied by a smooth, red, shiny tongue. If the patient has typhoid the tongue is pointed, red along the edges, with a thick coating in the middle. In malaria it is broad, thickly coated even at the edges, not sharply defined but filling the mouth like a piece of flaccid beefsteak.

Your tongue is needed for the process of eating as it shifts the food around and mixes it with saliva. When you swallow it presses against your teeth and the roof of your mouth so that food will be carried back and not forward.

Without your tongue you could hardly taste what you eat. The normal child is born with 328 taste buds on his tongue but after the age of 20 many tend to disappear and only about 100 remain. That is why children have such acute tastes and why people enjoy eating certain foods at one period and not at a later stage of their lives. The taste buds are connected with nerves which carry messages to centres of the brain which differentiate between enjoyment or distaste. That is also why children so hate bitter medicines and castor oil, dislike eating sago and greens like spinach, which their elders tolerate or even enjoy. That is why a ten-year old enjoys ice-cream three times as much as his grand-parents and revels in eating sweets. Taste buds enable the eater to differentiate between sweet, sour, bitter and salt.

Your tongue also denotes deficiencies in diet. A lack of *niacin* will make it scarlet, dry and painful, and sometimes bald and shiny; a lack of *riboflavin* will make it clean, shiny, magenta and the little nodules on its surface (taste-buds) will be atrophied and useless. A lack of *amino-acids* will make the tongue abnormally red; and iron deficiency, irritating and hot food will cause troublesome disorders of the tongue. It is not for nothing that for generations doctors have told patients to 'Put out your tongue', for it is one of the barometers of health. If you have chronic or recurring sores on your tongue, see a doctor without delay. See: Taste.

Touch. A sense which can produce either pain or pleasure. If something hot, pointed or sharp is touched the nerves nearest the skin at that point send their messages to the brain, which sends back an order to that part of the body to retreat; that is why you take your hand, for instance, sharply away from objects that burn, cut or prick. The sense of touch or feeling can be deceptive, however, for excitement dulls feeling temporarily. A hard knock suffered during a game of football, for instance, may pass unnoticed till the final whistle is blown, and there have been cases of men with broken legs playing on, for intense excitement can dull sensitivity. Where the body is badly burned Nature's defensive mechanism comes into operation and the shock is so great that no *pain* whatever, is felt at first. This often gives the doctor time to inject pain-killing drugs and relieve the victim.

The sense of touch can also be pleasant and stimulating and used judiciously, as in *massage,* can soothe and heal. See: Pain, Massage.

Trace Elements. Minerals so named because the merest traces are found in soils, which convey them in microscopic quantities into the stems, leaves, fruit and flowers of plants. If these elements are absent in soils certain diseases afflict those who eat foods grown in them; for instance, farmers in parts of Scotland, Denmark, USA, NZ and Australia noticed a peculiar disease afflicting cattle and sheep, which were stunted in growth, had poor coats, sunken eyes and lacked appetite. It was called 'daising' in Scotland, Denmark disease and 'grand traverse' in Michigan, and 'bush sickness' or 'Morton's disease' in New Zealand. Scientists set out to find the cause which was at first thought to be a lack of iron, but after 20 years it was discovered that the soil lacked cobalt.

Peach disease in California and citrus disease in Florida caused 'little leaf', and another hunt was started. Eventually these diseases were found to be caused by a lack of iron, for in Texas, where buckets of galvanised iron were used to keep the feed for trees, they were free from them.

The mineral content of soil differs widely. Once all farmland was covered by the sea, which on retreating left behind valuable minerals in the soil. Gradually the salt was washed away and foliage sprang into life, but heavy rain and floods leached away some essential elements in the course of millions of years, leaving poor soil in some areas. Once the 'impurities' in manures supplied the trace elements but with the almost universal use of concentrated fertilisers of 'high purity' these minerals are no longer added to the soil. The only way to ensure that the soil contains the 'trace elements' it needs – zinc, copper, manganese, boron, iron, cobalt, etc. – is to fertilise the soil with manures composted with straw, paper, and household wastes. See: Compost, Humus, Soil.

Tranquillisers. See: Drugs, Herbalism, Sleep, Valerian.

Turkish Bath. In principle much the same, but more elaborate than the *sauna.* The bather reclines in a room heated by steam, after which he is subjected to the ordeal of having cold water sloshed over him. Finally he is massaged vigorously and then allowed to rest or sleep. The idea is to rid the body of impurities through the pores by opening them with heat; then to prevent the risk of catching a chill by closing them with very cold water. The *massage* has the effect of breaking down minor lesions and producing a sense of well being and a loss of weight. Such baths should be taken only at long intervals, if at all, because they are apt to weaken the system. See: Sauna, Massage.

U

Ultra-Violet Rays. The so-called luminous rays of light are divided into three classes: (1) ultra-violet, below 400 millimicra (2) visible light from 800 to 400 millimicra (3) infra-red above one micron. Rollier, who probably had more experience than any other specialist in this field stated that during the early and late hours of the day sunlight has no ultra-violet rays. These can bring about an improvement in appetite, nutrition and the capacity for assimilating and metabolising food and an increase in well being and muscular strength. At the seaside these rays actually *increase* in strength when the sky is covered by light cloud, provided the sun is not hidden by cloud.

Excessive doses of ultra-violet rays can damage the skin and if concentrated by a sun lamp can be deadly. Eyes should be shielded by special dark glasses otherwise they can be irretrievably harmed and sight destroyed. No part of the body should be subjected to these rays for more than three minutes. The ultra-violet rays in sunlight must be treated with respect. According to Dr A. M. Kligmann, MD, of the Department of Dermatology, Pennsylvania School of Medicine, USA, sunlight and not innate ageing, is mainly responsible for the worst manifestations of shrivelled senile skin of so many Europeans and Americans who have laboured for years in the tropics; and the rays in sunlight which do most damage are the ultra-violet. See: Sunlight.

Ultrasonics. Ultrasonic (or supersonic) waves are those which range from 16,000 to 20,000 a second. During the last 50 years they have been harnessed to cure many diseases, allay pain and perform surgical operations: tonsillectomy, neuro-surgery and dentistry. Tumours have been removed by their aid, and they have benefited rheumatic sufferers and have been invaluable for pituitary radiation. In Russia where the science is well advanced, it has been found that ultrasonics give operators far more information than X-rays, for they make it possible, for instance, to see inside the eye and determine the anomalies of the crystalline lens. The science is in its infancy and is practised mainly by specialists trained in the subject and not by the ordinary GP. See: Vibrations.

V

Valerian (Valeriana officinalis). Only the root of the plant is used but it has many uses: in colics and fevers; for ulcerated stomach; and it is a powerful preventive of fermentation and gas. It is famous, however, as a valuable nerve tonic for it excites the cerebo-spinal system. It promotes sleep, conquers insomnia and is much valued in neuralgia, nervous debility and hysteria – especially when combined with scullcap. Insomniacs should boil one ounce in a pint of water for a minute, strain, and take a wineglassfull three times a day – one always before retiring. Larger doses before retiring usually have the opposite effect! See: Sleep, Drugs.

Van Pelt, Dr S. J. MB, BS. Former President of the British Society of Medical Hypnotists; Editor of the *British Journal of Hypnotism*; a member of the BMA; the National Association for Mental Health; the Society for Clinical and Experimental Hypnosis (New York); and The Society For The Study of Addiction to Alcohol and Other Drugs. Dr. Van Pelt, a pioneer in the field of therapeutic hypnosis, author of six books on the subject and co-author of three, had a specialist practice in London. He lectured widely, wrote numerous papers, articles for scientific journals on hypnotism, and was largely instrumental in elevating it from a form of stage entertainment to a scientific study. Most mental diseases and a variety of so-called physical diseases respond to hypnotic treatment. See: Hypnosis, Mesmer.

Vegan. One who lives on the products of the plant kingdom to the exclusion of flesh, fish, fowl, eggs or animal milk products. There are millions of vegans in India, and hundreds in Germany, Austria, America and Britain. Veganism is as much a matter of the indwelling spirit and mind as it is of a sound and balanced diet. Some vegans live exclusively on an all-raw food diet but most seek a balance between raw and cooked food. All lay stress on an abundance of fresh fruit, salads and nuts. The weakness of a vegan diet lies in a lack of calcium and the vitamins D and B$_{12}$ but this can be overcome if one knows how and those who wish to become vegans should ask the *Vegan Society* for further information and advice.

There are scientists who insist that man cannot live without animal *proteins;* but these are confounded by the abounding health of vegans who get their proteins from *yeast, nuts* and *seeds, legumes, soya* and other beans. *Calcium* exists in nuts, dried fruit, green leafy vegetables, plant milk, etc.

Vegan Society, The. Founded in 1944 for the promotion and dietetic education of vegans. The object is to provide in thought and practice for the advance of veganism and to relate veganism to every aspect of creative co-operation between Man and Nature. The address of the Society is: 47 Highlands Road, Leatherhead, Surrey.

Vegetarian. One who does not eat flesh or fish but lives on fruit, vegetables, nuts, beans, legumes, yeast and milk products. Those who feel it is wrong to kill animals, birds and fish for food find it easier, cheaper and more convenient to embrace vegetarianism than veganism. Most vegetarians eat eggs but the Jains, an Indian sect, will not touch eggs though they eat and drink milk products. Eggs, they maintain, are living animal organisms. Many vegetarians eventually make the transition to veganism.

There are cogent reasons for both veganism and vegetarianism: (1) compassion for all forms of animal life (2) health (3) preservation of the environment. Health reasons have the most practical importance, for though meat-eaters live as long as vegetarians, comparatively few enjoy advanced age without the afflictions of degenerative diseases such as arteriosclerosis, rheumatism and arthritis, diabetes, failing sight, and bladder and kidney diseases. The consumption of flesh foods is not harmful as long as the consumer remains active and is able to get rid of wastes through the pores, but as the elderly and old tend to discard hard physical exercise for a number of reasons, the accumulation of toxins usually takes its toll. *J. Ellis Barker* (not a vegetarian), wrote: 'I not only make all my patients vegetarians but I explain to them why I do so; and if they hesitate to accept my views I tell them that milk is liquid beef, that eggs are concentrated chicken, and cheese is beef in another form, etc.'

Drs Fisher and Fish say in *How to Live:* 'Meat-eating and a high protein diet, instead of increasing one's endurance have shown, like alcohol, actually to reduce it,' and they provide a number of examples from tests carried out on Yale students, athletes and instructors.

The *Report of the US National Conservation Commission*, Vol. III, p. 665, states: 'Comparative experiments on 17 vegetarians and 25 meat-eaters in the laboratory of the University of Brussels have shown little difference in superiority between the strength of the two classes, but a marked superiority of the vegetarians in point of endurance.'

Similar tests carried out by Professor *Russel H. Chittenden* at Yale had similar results. In every instance the endurance of vegetarian athletes was greater than that of those who ate meat.

Sir Hermann Weber, one of the Queen's physicians, who died at the age of 95 in full possession of his faculties, was not a vegetarian but was greatly in favour of a much reduced consumption of meat as one grew older. In *Prolongation of Life* he wrote: 'Many years ago I observed on myself that the reduction of the amount of food, especially meat and other flesh food, to half the quantity I had been in the habit of taking, enabled me to do a larger amount of work without the feeling of mental fatigue and exhaustion, and the craving for tea or coffee some hours after a meat meal.

'I have often succeeded in curing eczema, acne, roughness and scaliness of the skin and foetor (foulness of breath), by total abstinence during months and years from flesh, and the substitution of vegetables, especially green vegetables, milk, cheese and eggs in moderation. Not rarely this diet also led, as already mentioned, to great improvement of the complexion. It is worth mentioning that according to recent researches the vegetable albumins show a greater resistance to poisonous bacteria than animal albumins, and therefore are probably less prone to cause auto-intoxication.'

This view was endorsed by Dr C. Dukes in *The Bacteriology of Food*: 'Different types of microbes cause different kinds of decomposition of food, divisable roughly into two main varieties; fermentation due mainly to the decomposition of carbohydrates, and putrefaction due to the decomposition of flesh proteins. Whereas the products of the former are usually harmless, those of the latter are usually objectionable.'

Vegetarian athletes have proved that they are in no way inferior to those who train on meat. Indian wrestlers trained in the Akhara wrestling school of the vegetarian Guru Hanuman in Delhi, have won Olympic gold and silver medals. Other vegetarian gold medallists include Murray Rose, who created a world record; Tony Jarvis, who was appointed captain of Britain's Olympic swimming team; S. V. Bacon who won the Olympic Middleweight wrestling championship in 1908, the British Empire championship in 1911, and with his brother E. H. Bacon represented Britain in the Olympic Games at Stockholm and Antwerp. A list of their other achievements would occupy a page.

Paavo Nurmi, known as the Flying Finn, who won the 10,000 metres and 8,000 metres cross-country events and was second in the 5,000 metres at Antwerp, was the greatest of all vegetarian athletes. At Amsterdam he again won the 10,000 metres and in 1933 at the age of 36 the 1,500 metres in Finland.

For many years vegetarian swimmers and cyclists have proved that they are not inferior to flesh-eaters in stamina. *Eustace Miles* won the Real Tennis Championship of England ten times and that of the world once. Freddy Welsh and Eder Joffre were World Light and Bantamweight boxing champions respectively, events not generally associated with vegetarians; El Qufai won the Marathon in Amsterdam in 1928 and W. Kolehmainen won the Marathon in 1912 and held numerous world records between 25 and 26 miles. All were vegetarians.

Richard St Barbe Baker says that his grandfather, who was a great walker, once walked 42 miles before breakfast on a pint of beer, and was also a fine high and long jumper. Apart from health and ethical reasons vegetarianism makes sense as cereal and root crops that are fed to beef-raising animals could sustain many times the population they do, far more cheaply and with much greater benefit to health. The Irish peasantry who were tough, intelligent and long-lived, existed for generations (because they had to) mainly on potatoes; similarly, oatmeal was the staple food of the 'braw' Scots; and history tells us that the troops of Gustavus Adolphus and Charles XII of Sweden, who were invincible in their day, ate no meat whatever. (*Nutrition*: Dr W. F. Wernham).

Vegetarian, The New

The Vegetarian, official journal of the Vegetarian Society, was founded in 1848, a year after the Society was born. One of the founder members was Sir Isaac Pitman who invented the shorthand system bearing his name and it was under his imprint that it began, under the name *Vegetarian Messenger*. Later the London Vegetarian Society started *The Vegetarian News* which ran from

1920-1958, when the two periodicals were incorporated and called *The British Vegetarian*. In 1971 this was changed to *The Vegetarian*, which had a circulation of 55,000. In January 1977 the title was again changed to *The New Vegetarian* and was edited by *Mike Storm*, under whom it seemed to have a bright future as the number of vegetarians and vegans in Britain has increased considerably within the last two decades, for people are thinking more about their environment and the relations which should exist between humans and animals, which are being slaughtered, often in the most inhumane conditions, for food. The name of the magazine has now been changed to 'Alive'.

Venesection or Phlebotomy. The operating of cutting or opening a vein, as a medical remedy. A popular practice in the eighteenth and early nineteenth centuries, when men who could afford it ate and drank excessively and suffered from high blood pressure, hypertension and gout. Paracelsus and Ambroise Pare applied leeches to enlarged thyroids, which rapidly collapsed when blood was withdrawn from them, though this was only temporary. In some London hospitals leeches are still used to draw blood, but such methods are merely palliatives and do not affect the cause of the illness.

Vibrations. All matter is composed of vibrations, and the vibrations of the body in health differ from those in disease. *Sound, music, colour* and *speech* are the results of vibrations. Each article of food vibrates differently from all others; so do leaves and the petals of flowers. Vibrations can sooth and heal; they can also upset metabolism, create disease and destroy. Vibrations produce waves of different lengths and it is by knowing how these waves behave that we can harness them to produce health. The body also produces its own vibrations by the *emotions* created in the mind, which can bring health or disease, depending on the kinds of waves produced. See: Noise, Music, Colour, Speech, Emotions, Bach, Ultrasonics.

Virus. Derived from the Latin, slimy, liquid, poison. The virus, like the germ, is an agent of disease; not the cause. When you 'catch' a virus infection and your GP is baffled, he usually says: 'It's due to a virus' and sends you to hospital for observation.

Freidrich Loeffler discovered the virus in 1898 when he was searching for the cause of foot-and-mouth disease. He passed several tissues from diseased cattle through infusorial earth, the finest of filters, which removes all known bacteria. But when the filtrate was injected into healthy cattle they died. So he concluded that there must be a microscopic killer called 'virus', which till then was unknown. W. J. Elford, an Englishman, was the first to measure a virus. He found that it had a diameter of less than a millionth of an inch, and some viruses measure less than 30 millionths of a millimetre from end to end. The virus is smaller and more difficult to detect than any organism, and is far more resistant than the ordinary germ.

Professor R. G. Green, head of bacteriology at the University of Minnesota, says: 'They are the smallest units showing the reproductive property considered typical of life,' and the Ukranian scientist, Gorgei Gershenzon, that they change the heredity of micro-organisms, plants and even animals by disrupting the normal development of all systems. See: Bacteria, Microbes.

Vitamin. In 1881 Dr Lunin stated in a German scientific journal that 'substances other than casein, fat, milk, sugar and salts are indispensable for life.' Till then it was thought that milk, which contained these constituents, was a perfect food, but *Gowland Hopkins* in England, and McCollum, Osborne and Mendel in America were not convinced and in 1906 Hopkins said: 'No animal can live on a mixture of pure protein, fat and carbohydrates and, even when the necessary inorganic material is carefully supplied the animal still cannot flourish.' He maintained that an 'accessory substance' was necessary, and proved it in 1912. Dr Casimir Funk, a Pole, coined the word 'vitamine' to describe this substance, the first part *vita* relating to the life process, and the second to its chemical nature, because the original vitamine belonged to a group of substances known to chemists as *amines*. Later the 'e' was dropped and it was subsequently found that there was not only one vitamin, but many, and new vitamins are being found almost every year. Vitamins are not foods though they are found throughout the vegetable kingdom and in many animal products. Where processing has denuded foods of their vitamins their absence may be made up of vitamins in tabloid form, either natural or synthetic. See: Synthetic vitamins and Vitamins under the headings A, B, C, D, etc.

Vitamin A. There are three kinds of vitamin A: (1) that which is yellow in colour, exists mainly in the leaves of vegetables and is called carotene (2) that found in the livers of salt-water fish, known as A_1 (3) that found in the livers of fresh-water fish, known as A_2, A_1 and A_2 pass straight into the bloodstream and are absorbed. Carotene in green vegetables is acted upon by an *enzyme* contained in the human liver, which converts it into vitamin A. Unlike some vitamins, a lack of vitamin A rarely results in death though it is a common deficiency and can cripple and render the body ineffective. Nor is an overdose likely for the vitamin is not toxic unless more than 100,000 units a day are taken over a period of many months, and the daily requirements are not more than 6,000.

Vitamin A is soluble in fat but not in water and a lack of vitamin E in the body makes absorption difficult. A deficiency of A results in growth being retarded; teeth and gums will be malformed, and the conjunctiva of the eye, the linings of the respiratory, urogenital and digestive tracts become clogged and lifeless with horny cells. A lack also leads to eye troubles such as xerophthalmia and keratomalacia (night blindness), and even to deafness and tinnitus. Mineral oils such as liquid paraffin drain vitamin A from the body and in America one in every two persons suffers from a vitamin A deficiency. Vitamin A gives the skin a pink, healthy glow, keeps it free from wrinkles and protects the body from tumours. Stress also depletes the body of vitamin A.

The retina of the eye contains a pigment known as visual purple, composed of vitamin A and protein. When the eye is exposed to light this is converted to yellow, then white and some vitamin A is consumed in the process, and in the subsequent regeneration to purple when the retina is subjected to subdued light again. If vitamin A is lacking this conversion and regeneration is impaired and there is difficulty in seeing in glaring light, and again in a quick change to dim light after the eye has been subjected to bright light. Massive doses of vitamin A have also been given with success in cases of tinnitus and deafness.

This vitamin is found in butter, fortified margarine, fish oils, some fats, vegetable oils, pumpkin, carrot, spinnach, kale, broccoli, potato, sweet potato, parsley, peas, green and red peppers, paprika, olives, peaches, apricots and all green, leafy vegetables.

Vitamin B1. (Thiamin in America; Aneurin in Britain). Though originally it was thought that vitamin B was one substance only, it was found subsequently that there were many vitamins belonging to this family and even today more B-complex vitamins are being discovered, though we don't know all their functions. The first B-vitamin was isolated by Dr Casimir Funk, who started with 200 lb of yeast and by a process of elimination produced one-twelfth of an ounce of active material, so potent that one fifteen thousandth of an ounce cured polyneuritis in chickens. It was then given to humans with beri-beri and cured them. Beri-beri is virtually unknown in Britain as all but the poorest diets contain ample quantities of B$_1$ though a tendency to beri-beri has been found in some old age pensioners who cannot afford protective foods. Beri-beri starts with fatigue, a sensation of heaviness and stiffness in the calf muscles, inability to walk long distances and difficulty in breathing when walking upstairs. If the body is futher depleted of B$_1$ there will be headache, loss of appetite, dyspepsia, dizzyness, rough skin, a slow heart beat and diarrhoea alternating with constipation. A predominently refined starch diet causes these symptoms, but B$_1$ effects a rapid cure. The best sources of B$_1$ are brewer's yeast, wholewheat flour, soya beans, coarse oats, whole rye, ham, chicken, kidney, liver, pork, beans of every variety, all fresh and most root vegetables, peanuts and peanut butter. Milk and eggs contain a little B$_1$ and nuts and dried fruits contain traces. Excessive alcohol drains the body of this vitamin.

Vitamin B$_2$. (Riboflavin; also known as lactoflavin and vitamin G). Essential for growth and is part of one of the *enzyme* mechanisms through which food is burnt up in the body. Deficiency causes a disease known as *cheilosis* or *ariboflavinosis* which is characterised by a cracking and reddening of the skin at the corners of the mouth; lips and skin are abnormally red, there is a greasy feeling at the folds between nostrils and cheeks, and sometimes patients suffering from glare-blindness who do not respond to vitamin A will respond to B$_2$. Also all plant and animal tissues contain this vitamin, the best sources being yeast, wheat germ, milk, liver, eggs, cheese, leafy vegetables, soya and other beans, lentils, and the organs of animals. Baking, frying and roasting meats causes a loss of B$_2$; so does the boiling of milk and exposing it to strong sunlight.

Nicotinic Acid. (Niacin). In 1753 Casal reported a strange disease prevalent in Spain and in 1771 Frapoli named it *pelle agra* or roughened skin, but gradually it became apparent that there were other symptoms when pellagra appeared: pigmentation of the skin on the backs of the hands, face and feet, inflammation of the mouth, intense soreness and redness of the tongue, neuresthenia, anxiety, dizzyness, fatigue, numbness in parts of

193

the body, backache, headache, either constipation or diarrhoea, melancholia, depression and in the final stages, dementia. Eventually the patient is immobilized by cramp and eventually paralysis.

The disease was common in the Southern States of America among poor whites who lived on meat, maize and molasses and the symptoms were known as the three Ds – dermatatis, diarrhoea and dementia. Pellagra is not restricted to the United States but is found wherever maize forms the staple diet of the poor: Italy, Egypt, Romania and South Africa. In 1915 no fewer than 11,000 in the Deep South of America died from it; in 1917, 170,000 and in 1927, 120,000.

Then Dr Goldberger of the US National Institute of Health was sent to investigate the disease which was thought to be contagious but after many experiments he concluded that the cause was faulty diet. When he died in 1929 a cure had not been found. Not till 1937 when J. R. Madden at Wisconsin University extracted a crystalline substance called nicotinic acid from vitamin extracts was pellagra conquered. Now we know that nicotinic acid is contained in fresh vegetables, wholewheat bread, brewer's yeast, Marmite, Yeastrel, liver and liver extracts, fish such as salmon, herring and cod, wheat germ, almonds, brown rice, peanuts and a few other foods. It is now regarded as a member of the vitamin B family.

Vitamin B12. (Cyanocabalamin). The Ancient Chinese knew that the liver of birds and animals contained some substance that cured anaemia, but for pernicious anaemia there was no remedy. It was not till 1921 that Dr George Minot, an American, discovered that victims of pernicious anaemia also suffered from a wasting of the stomach. While on this research Dr Minot started to waste and was treated for diabetes and injections of insulin enabled him to continue his work. Dr Whipple, a colleague, then suggested that pernicious anaemia might be caused by the lack of some substance in the blood. In 1924 Dr W. Murphy persuaded patients with this disease to eat half a pound of raw liver and a quarter pound of raw meat daily and after two years 45 patients on this nauseating diet recovered. For this discovery Minot, Whipple and Murphy were jointly awarded a Nobel Prize for Medicine.

Further research was carried out mainly by Dr Mary S. Shorb and Dr Fokkers at the Maryland Agricultural Station in America and Dr Lester Smith and colleagues in Greenford, England, who claimed simultaneously to have discovered a missing factor, which they named B_{12} containing cobalt, as a cure for pernicious anaemia.

Vegetarians who object on principle to liver or liver injections need not be dismayed because Dr Selman W. Waksman, another Nobel Prize Winner, discovered that a mould called *Streptomyces griseus* is rich in B_{12} and can be manufactured at much less cost than B_{12} from liver, for it takes 20 tons of liver to produce one gramme of B_{12}. Dr F. Wokes, a vegetarian, found that vegans and vegetarians who have lived for years on a meatless diet are sometimes deficient in B_{12} after middle age, but B_{12} pills will rectify this. The human body is capable of absorbing only 4 microgrammes of B_{12} daily (a very small dose) and any excess is excreted from the body, so vegetarians should not be tempted to stuff themselves with B_{12} pills.

Vitamin C. (Ascorbic Acid). Scurvy is a disease which ravaged Northern Europe in the past for in winter fresh green vegetables and fruit were hard to come by. It was not until 1601 that it was discovered that lemons and oranges kept the disease at bay. Man, the primates and guinea-pigs are the only known animals to suffer from scurvy; cats, dogs, rats, rabbits and birds do not. Cows seem to have the ability to create vitamin C inside their bodies.

The first symptom of scurvy is roughness of the skin on the upper arms and thighs. Later, as the body is denuded of ascorbic acid gums grow painful and swell, teeth grow loose in their sockets, joints pain till every movement is unbearable, patches like bruising form all over the skin and there is a lack of stamina.

Ascorbic acid is the most unstable of all vitamins. Heat and exposure to sunlight tend to destroy it rapidly. So does excessive cooking, pressure cooking and the addition of bicarbonate of soda to boiled vegetables in order to preserve their colour. Cooking in copper or aluminium vessels also destroys the vitamin. Citrus fruit should be eaten as soon as the skin is cut or broken, and citrus juices and milk should not be left out in strong light.

There is considerable evidence to show that vitamin C protects the body against some forms of infection. Large doses injected into experimental animals increase antibodies (agents that combat bacteria) sevenfold. Dr Linus Pauling, winner of two Nobel prizes, claims that heavy doses of vitamin C, if taken in time will prevent colds and influenza, a point debated by medical men. However, even if it does not cure or prevent colds and flu there is no doubt that it provides increased resistance. The richest sources of vitamin C are grass and dandelions then come paprika, rose hips and *citrus fruit, berries, tomatoes, papaya*, water cress, mustard-and-cress, all green-leaf vegetables and *potatoes*. Most fruit other than citrus contain a little *ascorbic acid*.

It is not generally known that vitamin C is necessary for the formation of bone and the dentine in teeth, and it prevents tiredness.

Though the daily requirements of vitamin C are small, foods containing it should be eaten every day, but this should pose no problem if a balanced diet is eaten. See: Lind, Citrus fruit, Food reform.

Vitamin D. A lack of D causes rickets, once a chronic disease in British children, though it is prone to affect dark rather than light-skinned children. The vitamin was discovered only as a late as 1918, though for many years previously rickets had been cured by *cod-liver oil*. Lack of D results in a faulty deposit of *calcium* in the bones though not always in the teeth. If this calcifying agent is missing the bones grow soft and bend easily, causing bow-legs in young children, and other structural abnormalities.

Very little vitamin D is needed for health but as fruit and vegetables contain negligible quantities human needs must be met from eggs laid by hens fed on food containing cod-liver oil, and from butter, cheese, milk, herrings, mackerel, salmon, sardines, cod and halibut-liver oil, or from capsules containing them. There are 11 distinct types of vitamin D though the kinds concerning us are D_2 and D_3. D_2 is activated ergosterol which derives its name from the way it is manufactured; and D_3 is a substance present in animal fats. In 1924 it was known that rickets could be cured by (1) *sunlight* (2) *cod-liver* or halibut-liver oil (3) *ultra-violet rays* (4) food irradiated by ultra-violet rays. Finally, (5) it was discovered that this elusive element existed in sterols (waxy materials associated with fats in food) – but which? After innumerable experiments ergosterol (ergot-sterol, because it is derived from ergot, a fungus that grows on rye, and a sterol) was found to be the parent substance of vitamin D.

Very little is needed. One ounce of pure vitamin D is sufficient for a million doses! It is 400,000 times as potent as cod-liver oil and it is one vitamin of which the body can have too much; 500-1000 I.U. daily will prevent rickets; 1,000-3,000 will cure it;

100,000 is a toxic dose. Too much vitamin D given to babies will cause idiopathic hypercalcaemia, but normal doses aid and stimulate the healing of wounds. The safe dose for children is 1,000 I.U. and for adults 400-500 I.U.* Light and sunshine aid the formation of vitamin D in the body.

Vitamin E (Alpha Tocopheral – Beta Tocopheral). Vitamin E is found in more than 100 compounds, the most active being the *tocopherals,* derived from the Greek *tokos,* childbirth; *phero,* bearing, and *ol,* designating an alcohol. Discovered in 1922 by Evans and Bishop; in 1932 Evans and Burr released further information about it. They found, for instance, that if females were deficient in vitamin E they failed to reproduce, but if given E they could be cured; males deprived of E became sterile but the process could not be reversed.

Later the Canadians Dr E. Shute and Dr Vogelsang found that a deprivation of E affected the heart and feet and ankles swelled and grew painful. Doses of concentrated wheat germ oil reversed this process. E has also been found effective in phlebitis, varicose veins, muscular dystrophy and degeneration of certain parts of the eye due to advancing age. Dr Roger Williams, Director of the Clayton Foundation Biochemical Institute, University of Texas, says that a balanced diet containing six mg of E a day supplies enough vitamin E. The richest sources of E are wheat germ, wheat germ oil and corn oil. If 100% whole-wheat bread and flour products are always eaten instead of white bread and refined flour there is no need to take vitamin E supplements as these contain the germ of the wheat in which the vitamin exists. Flour of 85% or 81% extraction may not contain the germ.

Vitamins, Miscellaneous. New vitamins are constantly being discovered – mainly of the B-complex family; B_3, B_4, B_5, B_6 (pyridoxine), B_7, B_8, B_9, B_{10}, B_{11}, B_{13}, B_{14}, B_{15} (pangamic acid), B_c, B_p, B_t, B_w, B_x, H (biotin or coenzyme R factor), I, J, K (menadione, a blood clotting factor), L (casei factor), M, N, P (citrin eriodyctiol), R (coenzyme R factor), S (S. lactis factor), T, U, V, W, X, Y, pantothenic acid which is thought to be the same as B_3, *folic acid,* choline, inositol, para-aminobenzoic acid, rutin-bioflavinoids – hesperidin, anti-gizzard erosion factor, grass juice factor, etc. Research in these has been done on animals and not enough about them is known or about the way in which they affect humans.

* International Units.

W

Walking. A fine exercise for people of any age, which should never be made into a grim duty or penance. The old would be advised to perambulate gently. Some enjoy walking considerable distances, others do not. Never walk on when weary or exhausted. If no other exercise is taken, a walk every day is good for health; any distance from one mile to three.

Walking is one of the finest exercises for those who have suffered a stroke and are on the mend. They should walk gently at first and gradually increase the distance, but never strain their bodies. I know one man who had a stroke and now walks as far as ten miles at a stretch and never less than three or four miles every day.

If in normal health the middle-aged should walk upstairs rather than take a lift unless they are travelling more than five or six floors. But even a walk of ten floors will do them no harm.

Sufferers from varicose veins should take a brisk walk every day at a pace above normal.

Walking in gentle rain or in drizzle, provided you wear waterproof clothing, promotes health, for light rain or drizzle releases the negative *ions* so beneficial to health and has a wonderfully refreshing, tonic effect. Natives of countries like Britain and Ireland are fortunate in having so much light rain in which to walk.

Water, Drinking. If you weigh 150 lb 70% of your body, or 105 lb, consists of water. People have fasted for more than 200 days but no human can live for more than a week or ten days without water, which performs a number of functions in the body. It is (1) a constituent of all cells and tissues (2) the most important constituent of the blood (3) it acts as a solvent for food (4) a fluid medium for transporting and eliminating wastes (5) it carries waste products in the form of perspiration through the pores and out of the body, and as vapour through the lungs.

There is no hard and fast rule about the amount of water you should drink, which depends on temperature, dryness or humidity of the atmosphere, the kind of labour you perform and the kind of food you eat. A simple way of judging is by the colour of your urine. If dark and concentrated, you are not drinking enough; if lighter than straw (barring an indication of disease), too much. Normally vegetarians and vegans need less water than meat eaters and those who live on a heavy diet of carbohydrates, because raw fruit and vegetables contain distilled water in its purest form. Salt makes one drink far more than is necessary, but generally speaking, the best guide is thirst. Roughly about six pints a day is enough, including tea, coffee and soup. Salt foods, beer, wines and spirits, except in strict moderation, throw a strain on the kidneys. See: Hydrotherapy, Alcohol, Beer, Wine, Spirits.

Weight-Lifting. A form of exercise which has increased in popularity during the past 40 years. There are two kinds: (1) competition lifting in which the participant tries to raise more weight above his head in a specified manner than anyone else (2) weights used either for body-building or in order to excel in sport.

The first has little to recommend it for champion weight-lifters usually have monstrously distorted physiques, one or more parts, such as shoulders or chest, being out of proportion to the body as a whole. Weights used according to a system of progressive exercises, however, which develop groups of muscles, have much to recommend them.

The old idea that the use of heavy weights weakens the heart, is false. Weight training is as safe as any other form of exercise provided it is carried out under the eye of an expert. Weight training gives one an enlarged heart, says the critics, which is true. Great athletes have hearts larger than normal because the heart is a muscle, and like all muscles, grows bigger and stronger with constant heavy exercise. Beginners should start with light weights and increase, *very gradually*, to heavier ones. Never strain the body by handling weights that throw a severe strain on the limbs and heart.

During weight-training breathing should always be natural and unrestricted. Today sportsmen and women of every kind use weights in order to excel; not only boxers and wrestlers, but sprinters, tennis players, golfers, footballers, cricketers, high and long-jumpers, javelin throwers, hammer throwers and shot-putters. See: Exercise.

Wheat. Wheat is one of the oldest of the domesticated grasses and the staple carbohydrate food of the peoples of Northern Europe, America and North-West India. The wheat berry consists of an indigestible husk or outer protective skin; two other skins (bran); a glutinous substance called ceralin; a fourth layer

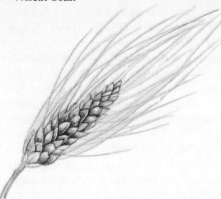

which can easily be digested; a fifth layer called aleurone composed of dark gluten cells (protein) and mineral salts; three more layers of starch cells; and near one end of the grain the straw-coloured germ, which forms about 2% of the berry. Any bread, flour or wheaten food which does not contain the germ is almost worthless, for the germ contains more than 50% of all the vitamins and is the only part that contains vitamins A and E. The whole grain consists of 13.40% water, 13.60% protein, 1.90% fat, 69.10% carbohydrates and 2.00% minerals, mainly phosphorus, potassium and magnesium. See: Bread.

Wheat Bran. See: Bran.

Wheat-Grass Therapy. Wheat-grass therapy is the result of years of experiment by Dr Ann Wigmore, author of *Why Suffer?* who has cured patients of innumerable diseases by making them chew wheat. Her ideas were enthusiastically embraced in India where during certain religious festivals the seeds of various plants, including wheat, are planted, each having a specific religious significance.

From ten to 20 leaves of the young plant are either chewed or the juice is extracted in some other way. This is done four times a day, the total amount of juice imbibed ranging from one to four ounces for patients suffering from chronic diseases. No other food is taken during treatment and the results, for those who persist, are said to be little short of miraculous.

Wheat grass may be grown at home in pots, from 10-30 grains in each pot, depending on the size. Only humus spread on garden soil, is used and no fertilisers of any sort should be added. If sprouted in a warm atmosphere the wheat should rise to a height of five-seven inches in from six to ten days. It should then be cut with a sharp knife or scissors and the roots pulled out, if the grass is allowed to grow taller than seven inches the juice is less effective; and if the juice is extracted by an electrical or mechanical grinder it should be sipped slowly immediately after extraction because after two or three hours it is valueless. Garlic juice may be added as a flavouring, but not lemon or salt. The quantities mentioned should not be exceeded as more than four ounces a day will cause nausea. The grass may be grown indoors or out, though it is advisable to grow it outside if the weather is warm.

In *Be Your Own Doctor* she claims astonishing success in curing dental troubles, pyorrhoea, most skin diseases, constipation, fatigue and lassitude, insomnia, indigestion and headaches; and other practitioners who have prescribed wheat therapy have succeeded in curing arthritis, skin allergies, grey and falling hair, stone in the kidney, failing sight, asthma, some kinds of paralysis, heart disease – even cancer and leprosy! It has also proved effective in reducing weight.

Wholewheat and Wholemeal. Wholewheat means 100% extraction, including the germ and bran. In wholemeal the extraction may be either 85% or 81%, with or without some of the bran and germ. Vegans, vegetarians and food reformers should always use wholewheat grown in compost. Sir Jack Drummond, official adviser to the Ministry of Health, said in *Englishman's Food* that there is some element in wholewheat which preserves teeth, but is lacking in other kinds of flour. Pies and tarts made from wholewheat, containing acid fruit, do not cause digestive troubles, whereas if other kinds of flour (especially white) are used, heartburn and digestive troubles are often experienced. Excellent pastry can be made from wholewheat, crisp and nutty in flavour.

Wiley, Dr Harvey W. After graduating from Harvard Medical School was appointed to the chair of Chemistry at Northwestern Christian University. After occupying several posts with distinction was made Chief Chemist to the Department of Agriculture in Washington, where he remained for 29 years. Renowned for his fight for pure food. He was the first to appoint 'poison squads' composed of volunteers, which he headed, to test suspect edibles on themselves. He did more than anyone in America to prevent adulteration of food, even going so far as to antagonise the leading manufacturers and bring down the wrath of President Theodore Roosevelt on his head. He feared no man and could not be bought. See: Saccharin, Preservatives, Processing, McCann.

Williams, Professor Roger J., MS, PhD. Born in India in 1893, the son of medical missionaries. When the science of nutrition was in its infancy he was teaching students at the University of Chicago about food and dietetics and writing his doctrinal thesis on yeast cells and their vitamin needs. He discovered *pantothenic acid* and did pioneer work on *folic acid*. Was the first biochemist to be elected President of the American Chemical Society. Received the Mead Johnson Award of the American Institute of Nutrition and since 1941 has been Director of the Clayton Foundation Biochemical Institute at the University of Texas, where more vitamins and their variants have been discovered than in any other laboratory in the world. He has played a substantial role in bringing our knowledge of nutrition to its present advanced state.

Wine. Wine has the sanction of the Scriptures. The Good Samaritan bathed the wounds of the victim who had been assaulted by robbers because it possessed antiseptic properties. In his Epistle to Timothy, Paul advised: 'Drink no longer water, but use a little wine for thine often infirmities.' Because of its health-giving properties, wine has been drunk by all civilised nations from the dawn of history and only when people drink immoderately or partake of adulterated wine, do they undermine their health.

Scientists who are not bigoted teetotalers have extolled the virtues of wine. Louis Pasteur said: 'Wine is the most healthful and most hygienic of all beverages.'

Dr Robert Steptoe, a Chicago obstetrician, stated that physicians should use more wine, which is one of medicine's most ancient remedies. A glass of wine is preferable to tranquillisers, pain-killers and drugs, which might easily disrupt a pregnancy. Furthermore, the effects of wine in small amounts must be largely psychological. If a glass of champagne can provide as much relief as a potent drug, we say choose champagne any time.'

In 1953 Dr Jan de Winter, consulting radiotherapist to the Brighton and Lewes group of hospitals, found that when patients were given doses of sherry during the diagnostic period the active lymph nodes could easily be located. They were then treated and were able to drink sherry with impunity and enjoyment.

In his *Treatise On Wine* Dr Thudicum wrote: 'We have never known an authentic case of *delirium tremens* produced by drinking, in whatever excess, natural wines.' Unfortunately most cheap wines (plonk) contain chemicals or are adulterated in some way.

The grape, both fresh and fermented, has some property not yet isolated, that is beneficial to the human body. Dr Johanna Brandt's *The Grape Cure For Cancer and Other Diseases* should be read by all who condemn alcoholic drinks outright. So should *The Grape Cure* by Basil Shackleton.

During a study of alcoholic beverages at Wisconsin University it was proved that wine does not injure germ plasma or have any hereditary influence. It neither hardens the arteries nor prevents hardening, and the idea that it corrodes the brain has no foundation. Nor is it a tonic and should not be taken 'to build up the body'. Taken in small quantities in the company of friends, wine is an excellent social habit.

A little wine in water of dubious quality makes it safer to drink. Canadian researchers have found that wine reduces the activity of a wide range of viruses that infect the human gut, chemicals found in the skin of the grape being responsible for the sterilising effect. They found that the concentration of these chemicals in the skin and juice of red wine to be ten times greater than of white, and also that polio virus was reduced to one thousandth of its strength by incubating it in grape juice for 24 hours.

One could fill a page with the names of octogenarians and nonogenarians who drank wine all their lives and were none the worse for it. Sir Moses Montefiore who lived to be 100 drank a bottle of port every day.

Jean Barotra, Wimbledon Singles Champion in 1924 and 1926, who is renowned for his vitality is still playing good class tennis at 78. In 1969 he played against an opponent 30 years younger during a tournament at the Queen's Club, London, and defeated him completely. When in 1952 he told the 27-nation Congress Against Alcoholism that sedentary workers should drink three quarters of a litre of wine daily and manual workers 1½ litres, he caused havoc and divided the delegates. But M. Andre Mignot, the Secretary, remarked: 'It's monstrous to forbid alcohol entirely. Next time we will have the delegates trying to prevent people from smoking and making love.' And Borotra added: 'It is ridiculous to talk about sinister influences. I have drunk wine in moderation all my life and the French members of the Congress know it'. See: Grape, Beer, Wine, Spirits, Alcohol.

Worsley, Professor J. R. President of the College of Traditional Chinese Acupuncture (UK); Leamington Spa; Professor of the College of Chinese Medicine (China); Master and Doctor of

Wrench, Dr G. T.
Acupuncture (China);
Hon. Professor of the
Department of Oriental
Medicine, Won Kway
University, Korea;
President of the Society
of the Advancement of
Traditional Acupuncture,
U.S.A.; President of the
Traditional Acupuncture
Society (UK); Consultant
to the Acupuncture Clinic,
Oaken Holt, Farmoor,
Oxford where, in
conjunction with his clinic
in Columbia, Maryland,
U.S.A., and the Clinic in
Leamington Spa students
are given experience
under Profesor Worsley's
supervision and the

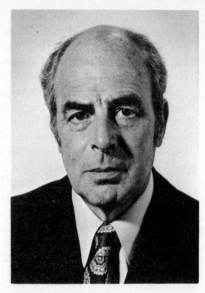

Professor J. R. Worsley

practitioners he has trained. Author of *Everyone's Guide To Acupuncture; Acupuncturist's Therapeutic Pocket Book; Is Acupuncture For You?* and *Meridans of CH'I Energy.*

Wrench, Dr G. T., MD, (London). A disciple of *McCarrison, Hindhede* and Sir *Albert Howard* and a pioneer into nutrition and soil research and their effects on health. Author of *The Wheel of Health,* one of the classics on nutrition, a volume that should be in every food reformer's library but which, sadly, is out of print.

Y

Yoga. Derived from the Sanskrit 'to yoke, join, make union with;' refers to a state in which action and thought are in complete harmony. There are branches of yoga to suit every person: *adhyata, bhakti, dhyana, ghatastha, hatha, kriya, laya, mantra, nana* or *jnana, raja* and *samkhya.* The more abtruse branches of yoga aim at the attainment of perception and intuition and are based on the results of trial and error over a period of centuries. The practical part of yoga consists of postures *(asanas)* and breathing *(pranayama)* of a kind peculiar to this philosophy. Their aim is the attainment of perfect health so that the student can forget the body and concentrate on the mind and spirit.

Yoga is not a religion. It is a complete philosophy which trains the mind to think and deal with the problems in life, and to develop powers of perception in order to realise the conscious-ness of the independent, self-existing, self-originating spirit of Man. It is ethical, embracing the science of human duty in its widest sense, and brings to the surface hidden powers. The intellect is developed through concentration and meditation; through constantly questioning and seeking answers so that the student becomes his own psycho-analyst and learns to solve any problem which may confront him, till eventually he achieves self-realisation which opens the gate to nirvana.

Yeast. The word yeast applies to numerous species in a botanical system of microscopic organisms, also known as fungi, which include *bacteria*. Pasteur is credited with being the first to study yeast cells and their division and discover the reason for their increase, though 50 years earlier Caginard de Latour studied yeast ferments in beer and described the living cells which reproduced by budding and attacked sugar in the process of growth. Later Dr Theodore Schwann, physician, physiologist and anatomist, established the organic nature of yeast.

Centuries earlier, however, it had been used to improve health and the Ebers Papyrus, inscribed in the 18th dynasty of Egypt (circa 1500 BC) recommended yeast as a cure for constipa-tion; and the Old Testament on several occasions mentions 'unleavened bread' made without yeast. Yeast has long been used for making both bread and wine and though the Ancients knew how it worked and what it did, they did not know why, or what it was.

There are two main types of yeast: wild and cultivated. The 'bloom' on grapes is wild yeast and is used in the fermentation process of wine-making; for most other purposes cultivated yeast is used, but it was not till 1870 that the scientist Hansen showed how it was possible to cultivate a pure strain.

The yeast cell closely resembles a hen's egg, though the egg is tens of thousands of times larger. It has a thin shell, an inner bark or membrane, albumen or white, and a yolk, embryo or nucleus. In analysis the constituents of the two are similar.

Food yeast or, as it is usually called, Brewer's Yeast, because it is one of the by-products of brewing, is a good source of high-class protein because it contains 17 amino-acids including the essential ones, and 17 vitamins, but negligible quantities of starch and fat. Casimir Funk found yeast to be one of the richest sources of B_2 and nicotinic acid. A quarter of an ounce of yeast a day sprinkled over salads, soups and other dishes is sufficient, and half an ounce is the maximum amount that should be taken. The body cannot assimilate more and if an excess is taken day after day a strain will be thrown on the organs of digestion and the kidneys and, according to Funk, W. G. Lyle and D. McCaskey the high purine content of yeast will raise the uric acid level of the blood and may lead to the formation of uric acid stones. As with most health-giving foods, a little is good for you but too much is harmful.

As the diet of many vegetarians – vegans in particular – is low in proteins, yeast makes a valuable addition to the diet and should not be neglected. For those who do not care for the slightly bitter taste, de-bittered yeast can be bought.

Constituents	Egg	Yeast
Proteins	14.80	12.67
Fat	10.50	0.80
Mineral matter	1.00	2.07
Water	73.70	73.80
Cellulose and other matter	—	10.66
	100.00	100.00

ACKNOWLEDGEMENTS

Individuals and institutions I have approached have, without exception, helped me freely with information and where possible, with pictures. I wish, therefore, to convey my gratitude and thanks to:

The Acupuncture Association, The Acupuncture Clinic, The Alfred Marks bureau, Mr. C. S. Allinson, The Allinson Co., Appleford, Mrs. Betty Bradbury, Mrs. Jo. Bradbury, Mrs. George de la Warr, Mr. Ian Miller of The C. W. Daniel Co., Mrs. D. M. Oxford, Mr. A. A. Lines of The Kellogg Co. of Great Britain, Mr. Peter Lief of Enton Hall, The Margaret Morris Movement, The British Homeopathic Association, The Biochemic Association, The Soil Association, Privatlink Bircher-Benner of Zurich, The Editor of *Prevention*, The Editor of *Here's Health*, The Schussler Biochemic System of Medicine, Carl Upton of The Psionic Medical Society, The Society of Teachers of The Alexander Technique, The British Chiropractic Association, The British Naturopathic & Osteopathic Association, Dr. G. Gordon, Mrs. Veronica Phillips, Dr. Barbara Latto, C. Leslie Thomson of the Kingston Clinic, Professor Hugh Sinclair, Kenneth and Angela Thompson, The Editor of *Alive*, Dr. Keki Sidhwa, Dr. S. J. Van Pelt, The Vegan Society, Professor J. R. Worsley, the Kirksville College of Osteopathic Medicine, Missouri, U.S.A., T. J. Wheeler, and Weidenfeld & Nicolson.